AF380086

COVID-19

From Basics to Clinical Practice

COVID-19

From Basics to Clinical Practice

Wenhong Zhang

Huashan Hospital of Fudan University, China

Translator-in-Chief: Xun Wang

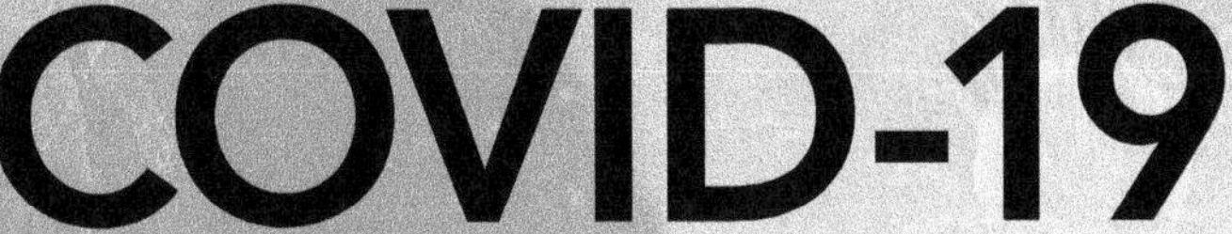

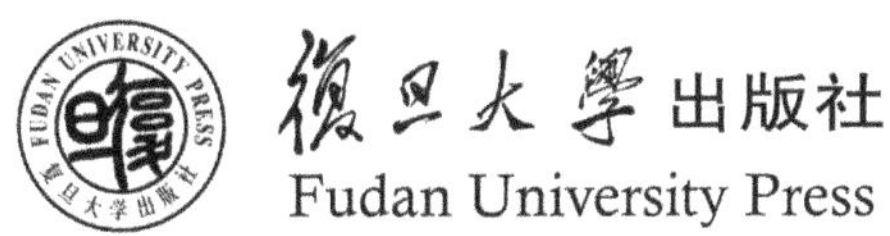

復旦大學出版社
Fudan University Press

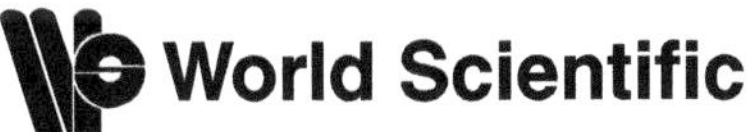

NEW JERSEY · LONDON · SINGAPORE · BEIJING · SHANGHAI · HONG KONG · TAIPEI · CHENNAI · TOKYO

Published by

World Scientific Publishing Co. Pte. Ltd.

5 Toh Tuck Link, Singapore 596224

USA office: 27 Warren Street, Suite 401-402, Hackensack, NJ 07601

UK office: 57 Shelton Street, Covent Garden, London WC2H 9HE

Library of Congress Control Number: 2020939566

British Library Cataloguing-in-Publication Data
A catalogue record for this book is available from the British Library.

《2019冠状病毒病—从基础到临床》
Originally published in Chinese by Fudan University Press Co., Ltd.
Copyright © Fudan University Press Co., Ltd. 2020
English translation rights arranged with Fudan University Press Co., Ltd.

COVID-19
From Basics to Clinical Practice

ISBN 978-981-122-206-1 (hardcover)
ISBN 978-981-122-207-8 (ebook for institutions)
ISBN 978-981-122-208-5 (ebook for individuals)

For any available supplementary material, please visit
https://www.worldscientific.com/worldscibooks/10.1142/11877#t=suppl

Desk Editor: Xiao Ling

Typeset by Stallion Press
Email: enquiries@stallionpress.com

Contents

Foreword

It was truly a herculean task for Professor Zhang Wenhong's team to compose this book, *COVID-19 — From Basics to Clinical Practice*, in such a short time.

To defeat an emerging infectious disease, what do we rely on? First, we rely on science. Second, we rely on participation: the participation of each individual, and the participation of the community. Third, we rely on trust: trust in ourselves, trust in healthcare workers, and trust in the government. During the battle against the epidemic, Wenhong not only actively treats patient day and night, but also spreads positivity to the general public through the media. He encourages people to participate, to believe in science, and to trust the government. He not only fulfills the due obligations of a physician, but also helps raise the awareness of public hygiene practices, as well as instills a better sense of responsibility in people.

During this COVID-19 pandemic, the boundaries among disciplines, universities, scientific institutions, and industries were broken for joint research. I hope to see more and more such stories of transitioning from "ownership by the entity" to "serving the people" in the future. Based on the established network of sentinel hospitals and pathogen monitoring stations in China, I suggest developing cross-disciplinary joint research models across the areas of veterinary science, human medicine, early warning systems, prevention, basic medical research, clinical practices, pharmacology, vaccinology, and traditional Chinese medicine. We should also establish a novel system for interdisciplinary and interinstitutional collaborations that are more open, coordinated, innovative, and cooperative. Such collaborations should not be transient, but rather represent the comprehensiveness and sustainability of the development in our infectious disease studies, and raise it to a new level.

I hope the publication of this book will be the starting point of new advances in this new discipline. I hope China can establish a more comprehensive and powerful system of basic research, control and prevention, as well as clinical treatment for infectious diseases. When another epidemic strikes, we will be better able to proactively and confidently take on the challenges, protecting the lives and well-being of the people.

Wen Yumei
March 15, 2020

Preface

Coronavirus Disease 2019 (COVID-19) is also known as Novel Coronavirus Pneumonia (NCP) in China. Like a sudden storm, it poses a serious test to China. In the face of this test, the community of infectious disease researchers in China further bears unimaginable responsibilities.

In December 2019, multiple cases of pneumonia with unknown etiology were reported in Wuhan, China. Because the pathogen behind it was not clear back then, and considering the main symptom being pneumonia, the disease was called "viral pneumonia of unknown cause". Later, it was confirmed that the disease was caused by a novel coronavirus, so its name was changed to "novel coronavirus pneumonia". However, with more understanding of this disease, it was found that the virus may not only cause pneumonia. Infected people can have no sign of pneumonia at all, while symptoms involving multiple other organs can appear. Meanwhile, the term "novel" is not suitable for naming a disease in a historical perspective. Therefore, the World Health Organization (WHO) changed its name to "Coronavirus Disease 2019 (COVID-19)" after much discussion.

Following the emergence of the disease in Wuhan, the epidemic rapidly spread via the movement of the population throughout Hubei province and the rest of China. The disease has subsequently appeared in other countries in Asia, Europe, North America, and Oceania, evolving into a storm still sweeping the globe to this day. The main features of this disease are the extremely high transmissibility and fast progression in some patients. The disease quickly spread in only a few months. By February 29, 2020, the global cumulative number of confirmed cases reached 84,607 with 2,914 deaths; in mainland China, the cumulative number of confirmed cases reached 79,251 with 2,835 deaths. China was facing a daunting task, and now the world faces the same.

The current pandemic shares some commonality with, but also is different from, the H1N1 influenza pandemic in 1918 and the Severe Acute Respiratory Syndrome (SARS) epidemic in 2003. All were caused by a hitherto unknown respiratory infectious disease, which then spread globally. Additionally, because the entire population lacked immunity, all three viruses resulted in huge casualties. Unlike the outbreak either 100 or 17 years ago, when the current epidemic emerged, the world now is more globalized, with transportation and traveling more convenient. These have led to a far wider and faster spread of disease than before. At the same time, since COVID-19 is caused by a different pathogen than the ones behind influenza and SARS, their pathogenic and epidemiological characteristics are not the same.

Humanity's fight against emerging infectious diseases calls for global collaboration and mutual support. The experiences and research findings accumulated during the global fight against this plague should be shared as quickly as possible. In less than two months, the achievements of Chinese scientists have attracted worldwide attention; never has any research community made such substantial research progress in such a short time on an emerging novel infectious disease. The progress includes identifying the disease-causing pathogen, sequencing and sharing its complete genome with the world at the earliest possible time, specifying preliminary routes of transmission, determining the incubation period and clinical characteristics of the disease, clarifying the survival time of the virus in the environment and its sensitivity to varying disinfectants, establishing laboratory tests for rapid diagnosis, and summarizing preliminary plans for effective treatments.

It is noteworthy that the healthcare workers in China have had a plethora of experiences with the epidemiology, clinical treatment, and prevention of COVID-19. To cope with the shortage of medical staff in Wuhan and the entire Hubei province during the epidemic, Fudan University Affiliated Huashan Hospital sent 273 medical professionals in five groups to the area, in addition to the tens of thousands of medical professionals from all over the country. Some of them worked at hospitals that exclusively managed serious and critical patients, while the rest worked at the Fangcang shelter hospitals receiving infected patients with mild symptoms. They fought alongside the local medical staff on the frontline against COVID-19, saving the lives of a great number of infected people and preventing further spread of the disease. Their experiences have been shared through publications in both domestic and international scientific journals. These accounts provided valuable information and guidelines for clinicians across the country in diagnosing and treating the disease. The physicians, medical experts, and academy fellows fighting on the frontline also shared their invaluable experiences on its prevention and treatment through various media on different occasions, providing enormous support to other medical practitioners across China.

Now that the battle against COVID-19 is in full swing globally, substantial advances have been made in the understanding of its etiology, epidemiology, diagnosis, and therapeutics. It is high time that we, as one of the first groups of medical practitioners fighting against COVID-19, compile the current progress and outcomes achieved in the global fight against the disease. To this end, we gathered frontline experts from the Department of Infectious Diseases, Huashan Hospital, who have been working long term in the fields of clinical infectious diseases, basic medicine, and hospital infection control. Our team ploughed through a considerable body of literature on COVID-19, and learned about the field experiences of Chinese healthcare professionals. In this book, we strive to recapitulate what is known about COVID-19, from basic research to clinical prevention and treatment. By publishing this book, we hope to help interested readers understand research advances on its treatment and prevention.

It is particularly worth mentioning that, as the head of Shanghai's COVID-19 clinical expert team, I collaborated with experts from other major hospitals in Shanghai to jointly work at the Shanghai

Public Health Clinical Center. Within slightly over a month, we have successfully treated more than 300 COVID-19 patients. We have also summarized our experience in "Comprehensive Treatment and Management of COVID-19: Expert Consensus Statement from Shanghai", which is published in the *Chinese Journal of Infectious Diseases*. We have referenced part of the expert consensus when composing this book, and hence included its full text as an appendix at the end of this book for readers' references.

Furthermore, together with my colleagues at the Department of Infectious Diseases, Huashan Hospital, we composed more than 20 science communication articles regarding COVID-19 through the "Huashan Infectious Diseases" WeChat social media account during the outbreak. In these articles, we analyzed the epidemic situations, evaluated tentative strategies for prevention and control, and publicised scientific knowledge on the correct preventative measures. Collectively known as "The Battle Diary", our communication articles were widely welcomed and well received by the online readers. In less than two months, each article garnered nearly or over 100,000 reads on average; some even attracted more than one million readers.

With the rapid advances of current research on COVID-19, an increasing number of new studies are being published every day. Due to the limitations both in time and in the authors' experience, errors and omissions are inevitable. We look forward to feedback from peers and readers to further improve this book and update our understanding of the disease for future editions.

The COVID-19 pandemic is still raging when this book goes to press. We whole-heartedly thank the experts and scholars fighting on the frontline against COVID-19, whose first-hand experiences with disease prevention and treatment make this book truly valuable. We are also grateful to the experts in basic medical and epidemiological research on COVID-19. The research results from their unceasing efforts allow this book to reflect the latest advances in COVID-19 studies.

Finally, we look forward to a speedy conclusion in the fight against COVID-19. We wish all our peers triumph in this war and a safe return to their families.

Zhang Wenhong
Shanghai, February 29, 2020

List of Contributors

All of the contributors are from Huashan Hospital of Fudan University, China:

Acknowledgments

The publication of the English version of this book is funded by the Morningside Foundation.

We especially thank the following people and institutions for the translation and publication of the English version of this book:

- Professor Zhang Wenhong and his team for granting the copyright to the English version free of charge and reviewing the translation.
- Di Jianzhong (Shanghai Jiao Tong University Affiliated Sixth People's Hospital) and Liu Qihui (Fudan University Affiliated Huashan Hospital) for proofreading the translation.
- Thirteen voluntary translators for translating this book into English free of charge:

Wang Xun (Translator-in-Chief)
PhD degree in Biomedicine from Karolinska Institutet;
Vice President of China Sweden Life Science Association,
Stockholm, Sweden

Cheng Xiaoheng (Team Leader)
PhD candidate in MCIBS (evolutionary genetics),
Pennsylvania State University, USA

Qin Zhizhen (Team Leader)
Translator and interpreter, graduated from Beijing Foreign Studies
University, China

Yuan Rongjie (Team Leader)
Lecturer in interpreting and translation, East China Normal University, China

Cheng Siyuan (Lily)
Graduate student, Department of Genetics, Yale University, USA

Ding Ruoyu
Student, School of Social Development, East China Normal University, China

Li Haiqi
Student, Cambridge School of Weston, USA

Luo Chuqiao
Graduate student, Department of Breast Surgery, Fudan University Shanghai Cancer Center, China

Nie Yao
Intensivist, Department of Critical Care Medicine, the First Affiliated Hospital of Sun Yat-sen University, China

Xin Chao
Student, Shanghai International Studies University, China

Xue Bing (Grace)
Senior translator at HCRDI, China

Yang Xuejiao
Translator and interpreter, CRRC Qingdao Sifang Rolling Stock Research Institute Co., Ltd., China

Zhang Yi
Translator, graduated from Sun Yat-sen University, China

Fudan University Press

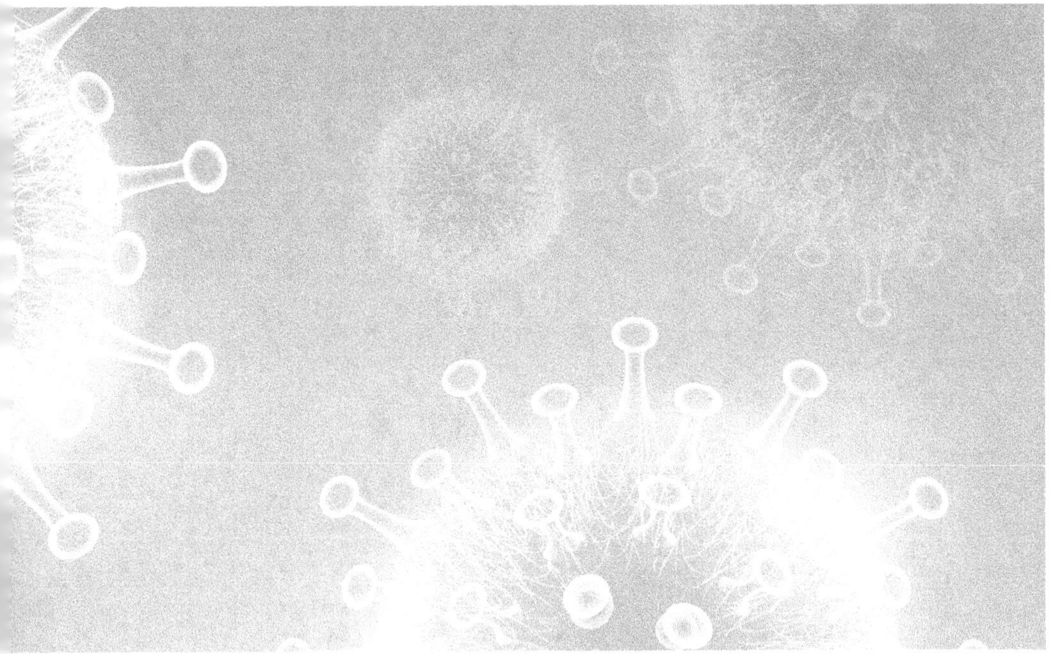

Part 1

Epidemiology

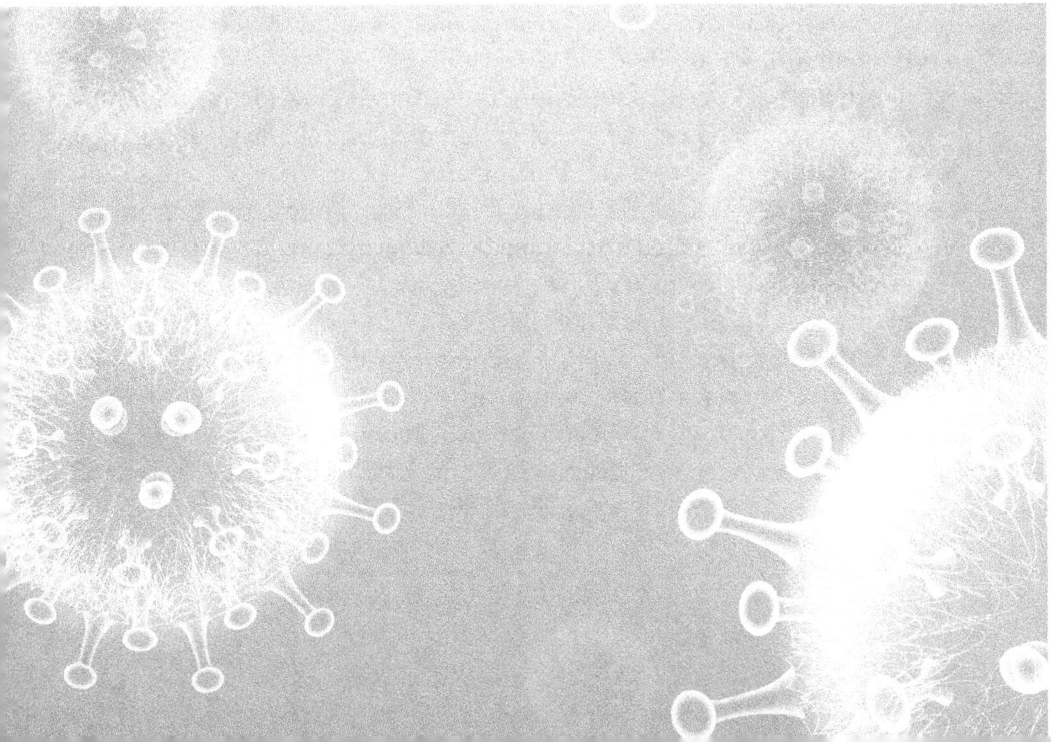

Chapter 1
Epidemiology Review

1.1 Naming the Disease and Its Pathogen

Coronaviruses are a family of viruses found in animals and humans. Some can infect humans and cause common cold or more severe diseases such as Middle East respiratory syndrome (MERS) and severe acute respiratory syndrome (SARS).

The novel coronavirus was first isolated and identified at the end of 2019 and the beginning of 2020. This emerging pathogen was confirmed to be entirely new to human history. In less than three months, both the naming of the virus and the description of disease characteristics have changed many times, as understanding on these deepened.

In early January 2020, before the pathogen was identified, China initially called the disease "viral pneumonia of unknown origin" due to its main symptom of inflammatory pulmonary changes. On January 7, 2020, Chinese Center for Disease Control and Prevention (China CDC) isolated the strain of the virus and identified it as a novel coronavirus (nCoV). The disease was thus renamed "pneumonia caused by the novel coronavirus". On January 30, the World Health Organization (WHO) recommended "2019-nCov" as the respective interim names for the virus and disease. On February 8, National Health Commission of the People's Republic of China (PRC) announced the decision to temporarily name the disease as "novel coronavirus pneumonia", or NCP.

On February 11, the *Coronaviridae* Study Group of the International Committee on Taxonomy of Viruses (ICTV) officially named the virus SARS-CoV-2. On the same day, WHO announced the name change of novel coronavirus pneumonia to "coronavirus disease-2019", abbreviated as COVID-19 (COronaVIrus Disease-2019), with 2019 standing for the year that the first case was seen. This decision is based on the consideration that the infected patients can experience a wide range of clinical manifestations, from no symptom to severe or critical condition presenting with not only lung injury, but also multiple organ function lesions. Therefore, it is inappropriate to name the disease pneumonia.

Although there is still controversy over their names, we will use SARS-CoV-2, named by ICTV, and COVID-19, named by WHO, as the virus and disease names, respectively, for the remainder of this book. However, direct quotations from related literature are kept without changes.

1.2 Overview of the Epidemic in China

1.2.1 *Early cases and transmission*

The first cases in China were reported in the city of Wuhan in Hubei province. In December 2019, some medical institutions in Wuhan received patients with unexplained bilateral pulmonary infiltrative lesions in chest radiographs. Many of these patients had visited a local seafood wholesale market where some vendors sold wild animals such as masked palm civets, bamboo rats, and snakes. With swift development in identifying the pathogen and tracing the virus, it was later confirmed that these patients with unexplained pneumonia were infected by a novel coronavirus. Subsequent epidemiological investigations indicated a regional outbreak of COVID-19 in December 2019, in which the earliest cases dated back to the beginning of the month. There could already be patients who had onset of the disease prior to the outbreak, and super-spreading incidents occurred in the seafood market soon after. In conclusion, the early epidemiological tracing played a crucial role in confirming the source of the virus.

According to a retrospective study by Epidemiology Working Group for NCIP Epidemic Response of China CDC, the total number of COVID-19 cases had risen to 104 as of December 31, 2019, distributed in 14 counties and districts in Hubei province. In other words, at this early stage, the virus had already silently gone rampant across Hubei before people found out about this "adversary". On December 31, Wuhan authorities concluded their preliminary epidemiological studies and closed the seafood market on January 1; meanwhile, the outbreak had developed into the second stage.

1.2.2 *Stages of community transmission*

In early January, the virus spread rapidly, marking the second stage of the outbreak — community transmission. Patients exposed to the seafood market in the first stage spread the virus to the community, leading to large-scale interpersonal and clustered transmissions across households and communities in Hubei. Studies suggested that the proportion of cases associated with the seafood market in Wuhan decreased significantly from 55% to 8.6% before and after January 1, 2020 respectively.

After ruling out known respiratory pathogens such as human influenza viruses, avian influenza viruses, adenovirus, SARS coronavirus (SARS-CoV), and MERS coronavirus (MERS-CoV), the pathogen was identified as a novel coronavirus. On January 7, 2020, this novel coronavirus was isolated and its whole genome sequences were subsequently acquired. Nucleic acid-based assays detected 15 positive cases, and the morphology of coronaviruses was revealed on a sample isolated from one positive patient under electron microscopy. WHO later commented, "Preliminary identification of a novel virus in a short period of time was a notable achievement and demonstrates China's increased capacity to manage new outbreaks". This was much faster than identifying the pathogen during the SARS outbreak.

Due to the underestimation of the virus's interpersonal transmissibility in the early stages, the number of cases grew exponentially. According to retrospective studies, 566 cases showing symptoms were recorded in Hubei province from January 1 to 10; during the same period, 87 cases were found in 19 other provinces and municipalities including Henan, Chongqing, and Hunan. This indicated that the epidemic had spread to the whole country. However, only 41 cases had been diagnosed nationwide (all in Wuhan) as of January 10.

Following the start of the Spring Festival travel season, COVID-19 progressed into the third stage — the large-scale spread of the epidemic. During this stage, a surge of primary and secondary cases hit Hubei province. Meanwhile, a large number of infected patients traveled across the country and imported cases emerged in other municipalities. On January 19, the first cases of infection among healthcare workers were confirmed, demonstrating coronavirus transmission between humans. On the same day, National Health Commission of PRC reported the first imported case of COVID-19 in Guangdong province, which represented the first reported case outside Hubei in mainland China. The following day, another five cases were reported in Beijing and two in Shanghai. National Health Commission of PRC received reports of 291 confirmed cases as of January 20, of which 270 were in Hubei. In retrospect, there were a total of 5,417 cases with symptoms from January 1 to 10 nationwide, including 4,121 in Hubei and 1,296 outside of Hubei. On January 20, following the approval by the State Council, the National Health Commission decided to classify COVID-19 as a Class B infectious disease as stipulated in the *Law of the People's Republic of China on the Prevention and Control of Infectious Diseases*, and to adopt measures for prevention and control as if it was a Class A infectious disease. They also listed it as among quarantine-restricted infectious diseases stipulated in the *Frontier Health and Quarantine Law of the People's Republic of China*. Provinces and municipalities immediately mobilized their emergency responses. From January 20 to 23, 25 provincial-level regions reported newly confirmed cases of COVID-19. The total confirmed cases in 29 provinces and municipalities reached 830 as of January 23. Fourth generation infection cases were reported, suggesting sustained interpersonal transmission of the virus.

COVID-19 patients are contagious during the incubation period, so it is far more difficult to conduct epidemic prevention and control than SARS; in addition, the epidemic also peaks faster. Henan province reported a cluster of cases caused by family gatherings. Patient A, a 20-year-old female, lived in Wuhan and visited the city of Anyang in Hunan on January 10, 2020. From January 10 to 13, She had contact with five local relatives (patients B-F). After one of them started to show symptoms of COVID-19, patient A was quarantined and closely monitored. As of February 11, her temperature had been normal and she had neither self-reported fever nor gastrointestinal or respiratory symptoms (including cough and sore throat). On January 27, her CT scan was still normal but she was confirmed to be infected with SARS-CoV-2 the next day. Before then, however, the other four relatives were all diagnosed as having COVID-19. Considering patient A's timeline and the absence of other epidemiological links to Wuhan among her five relatives, she could be a case of asymptomatic super spreader. A study on 72,314 confirmed cases suggested 1.2% of the people infected were asymptomatic, which is not a substantial fraction. Further studies are needed to investigate the infectivity of asymptomatic carriers and that of people in the incubation period.

1.2.3 *After implementing containment measures*

On January 23, 2020, Epidemic Prevention and Control Headquarters of Wuhan imposed lockdown laws, including the suspension of the city's buses, subways, ferries, and long-distance passenger transportation, as well as temporary closure of the departure channels of airport and railway stations. By the following week, other cities and provinces also implemented traffic restrictions. From January 24 to 28, people with COVID-19 entering other cities and provinces before the Wuhan lockdown started developing symptoms, pushing the epidemic to its first peak. A cumulative total of 32,642 COVID-19 cases developed signs and symptoms before January 31 in mainland China, distributed across 1,310 counties and regions. Of these cases, 74.7% was in Hubei. Meanwhile, China's National Health Commission received reports of 11,791 confirmed cases in mainland China, of which 60.7% was in Hubei. Since then, except for the spike reported on February 1, the number of reported cases has been steadily declining. The epidemic outside Hubei province has been effectively curbed

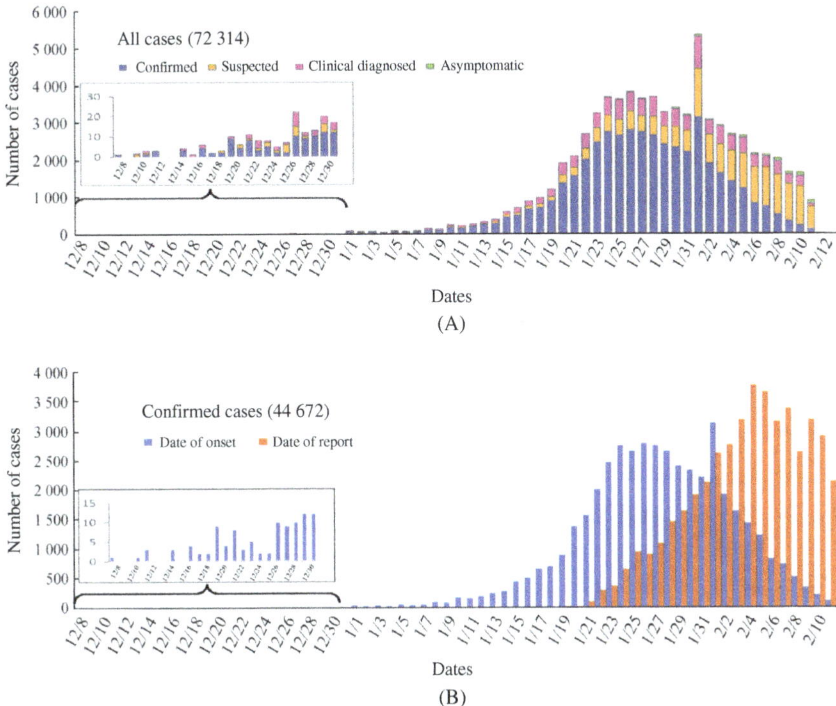

Figure 1-1. Confirmed COVID-19 cases as of February 11, 2020. **A**: Epidemic curves of COVID-19 confirmed, suspect, clinically diagnosed and asymptomatic cases reported in mainland China; **B**: Epidemic curves by symptom onset and date of report for confirmed COVID-19 cases for mainland China (Cited from: Epidemiology Working Group for NCIP Epidemic Response. The epidemiological characteristics of an outbreak of 2019 novel coronavirus diseases (COVID-19) in China. [Chinese]. *Chinese Journal of Epidemiology.* 2020;41(2):145–151.)

with the implementation of prevention and control measures such as travel restrictions and social distancing.

The number of reported cases nationwide peaked on February 5 but has been slowly declining since then, with the number outside Hubei province steadily decreasing (Figure 1-1). As of February 19, there were a total of 74,576 confirmed cases reported in mainland China, of which 62,031 were in Hubei province (45,027 in Wuhan). Sixty-five confirmed cases, including five deaths, had been reported in the Hong Kong Special Administrative Region (SAR), 10 confirmed cases in the Macao SAR, and 24 with one death in Taiwan. Among them, five patients in Hong Kong, six in Macao and two in Taiwan had been discharged from hospitals after recovery. At this stage, more characteristics of COVID-19 emerged, such as the rate of serious illness and the case-fatality rate (CFR). According to literature published at the early stage of the outbreak, the rate of serious illness ranged from 15% to 25% and the crude CFR from 2% to 3% in mainland China.

The crude CFR in Hubei Province (2.9%) was significantly higher than that in other provinces (0.4%). CFR dramatically increased once patients progressed to severe or critical stage compared to patients with mild or moderate illness. According to previous studies, the crude CFR of critically ill patients reached 49%.

As of February 28, the epidemic in China has been declining overall but has not yet ended. Current measures of high-level emergency responses should continue after the resumption of work and production because the risk of COVID-19 transmission increases due to large volume of human traffic and interaction, while social distancing becomes less feasible.

After investigating China's prevention and control measures, as well as epidemiological studies, WHO assessed that the radical intervention of "whole-government, whole-society" had probably prevented at least tens of thousands of COVID-19 cases. Typical epidemic models of infectious disease outbreak expect the number of total infections to continually go up and peak, followed by an extended plateau, before eventually go down, until susceptible individuals are few enough to curb further transmissions. However, the curve in China has a plateau-like high point before sliding down. In epidemiology, such shapes often occur because of the progressive and effective measures taken by policy makers to educate and guide the public. Examples of such measures are travel restrictions and home quarantine orders.

From February 10, 2020 onward, areas outside Hubei province gradually started lifting restrictions to reopen the economy and restore pre-epidemic social orders. With barely any new cases of COVID-19 being detected and the economy recovering, it is critical to phase the lifting of various restrictions. At the same time, extreme caution should be exercised to carefully manage the risk of the virus reimporting and resurging as restaurants and shops reopen and schools restart. Only through this route can the country safely, albeit slowly, gets back on its feet after the rampage of this epidemic. Even afterward, alertness should be maintained in detecting new cases.

1.3 The Epidemic Outside of China

1.3.1 *Overview of the epidemic outside of China*

Since mid-January 2020, other countries have been reporting confirmed COVID-19 cases one after another. On January 13, a visitor from Wuhan was diagnosed with COVID-19 in Thailand, becoming the first case outside of China. On January 21, the United States reported its first imported case, marking the first outside of Asia. On January 31, WHO declared the COVID-19 outbreak a Public Health Emergency of International Concern (PHEIC) because of the rise in cases in both China and other countries.

As of February 28, 2020, according to data on WHO's website, 4,691 COVID-19 cases were reported across 51 countries, territories, and areas outside of China, covering Asia, Europe, the Americas, Oceania and Africa. Among them, more than 50 cases were reported in six countries and areas, of which 2,337 were in South Korea, 210 in Japan, 705 on the Diamond Princess cruise ship, 650 in Italy, 245 in Iran, 96 in Singapore and 59 in the US. Over ten deaths were reported in three countries and areas, of which 26 were in Iran, 17 in Italy and 13 in South Korea. As of the completion of this book, the number of new cases is still rising rapidly in some countries.

On February 28, Director-General of WHO Dr. Tedros Adhanom Ghebreyesus announced in Geneva that the threat assessment for COVID-19 was elevated from "high" to "very high", its highest level. "The continued increase in the number of cases, and the number of affected countries over the last few days, are clearly of concern," said Dr. Tedros. "We have now increased our assessment of the risk of COVID-19 to very high at a global level." He noted that the global prevention and control of COVID-19 has entered a "decisive moment". WHO further advised that every country must take robust action to prepare for all possible scenarios, and that no country should gamble on having no cases imported. He added that, "[o]ur greatest enemy right now is not the virus itself. It's fear, rumors, and stigma." On the same day, António Guterres, Secretary-General of the United Nations, stated at the United Nations headquarters, "[w]e know containment is possible, but the window of opportunity is narrowing." He urged that all governments should step up together and do everything possible to contain the disease.

With respect to the development of the epidemic, the key to prevention and control is to contain local transmission within every country and territory. These results rest on various factors including the timing of warnings, risks of local viral transmission, local healthcare systems and resources, governments' execution of policies, and public compliance. As of end February 2020, the number of new confirmed COVID-19 cases is still rapidly increasing in some countries, and the development may well go any direction.

1.3.2 *The outbreak on the Diamond Princess cruise ship*

Most confirmed COVID-19 cases in Japan were from the Diamond Princess cruise ship. On January 20, 2020, the cruise ship departed Japan. On January 25, a passenger developed a fever after disembarking in Hong Kong, and was tested positive for COVID-19 on February 1. Two days later, the ship urgently returned to Japan and all the people on board were quarantined in the ship for two weeks from February 5, with passengers confined to their cabins. Limited by the shortage of test kits, Japanese authorities could only run nucleic acid tests for the virus on a small proportion of passengers. Meanwhile, conditions on the cruise ship rapidly deteriorated due to the lapses in epidemic prevention and control measures on board. As of February 12, 492 passengers were tested and 174 were diagnosed with COVID-19, including one Japanese health official responsible for testing passengers. On February 19, the day when the 14-day on-board quarantine was supposed to end, testing for all people on board was finally completed, and the number of confirmed cases rose to 621, much higher than the number in Shanghai then. As of February 28, 705 people had the disease. The Diamond Princess cruise ship became the first site of a large-scale COVID-19 outbreak outside of China.

Notably, four deaths have already been reported among the confirmed cases. The outbreak on the Diamond Princess cruise ship became a highly educational event in the history of emerging infectious diseases, providing valuable lessons for their prevention and control, not only during that time but also in the future. First, everyone is susceptible when a novel infectious disease strikes because the population has not establish effective immunity against it, and no one will be spared if no intervention is implemented. Second, controlling an outbreak is premised on identifying the source of transmission. The most critical first week of window of opportunity for on-board quarantine and testing was missed, resulting in the continuous spread of the virus. Moreover, the quarantine on the Diamond Princess cruise ship mainly prevented exporting cases to the outside but did not completely solve the problem. In fact, only when the quarantine of each person is enforced can the transmission be stopped. Traffic restrictions without individual quarantine means the epidemic will continue to spread.

Chapter 2
Epidemiological Characteristics

2.1 Sources of Transmission

At present, SARS-CoV-2 patients are the primary source of transmission. Asymptomatic infected individuals could also be a source of spread of the novel coronavirus. Further studies and research are required to investigate the infectivity of people during the incubation period and convalescent patients.

2.1.1 *Origin of the virus*

SARS-CoV-2 belongs to the genus *Betacoronavirus*. SARS-CoV-2 is most closely related to the bat SARS-like coronaviruses derived from Chinese horseshoe bats (*Rhinolophus sinicus*), with a nucleotide sequence homology of over 85%. It has a 78% nucleotide sequence homology with the human SARS-CoV, while differing greatly from MERS-CoV with a nucleotide sequence homology of merely 50%. Researchers obtained complete genome sequences from five patients during the early phase of the epidemic. Their genome sequences were almost identical and had a 79.6% nucleotide homology with SARS-CoV. Moreover, the analysis on the full-length genomic sequence showed that SARS-CoV-2 was highly similar to Bat-CoV-RaTG13, which was previously detected in Chinese horseshoe bats from Yunnan province, with an overall genome sequence identity of 96.2%. Though further analysis indicated that the full-length genome sequence of SARS-CoV-2 shared less than 80% nucleotide sequence identity with

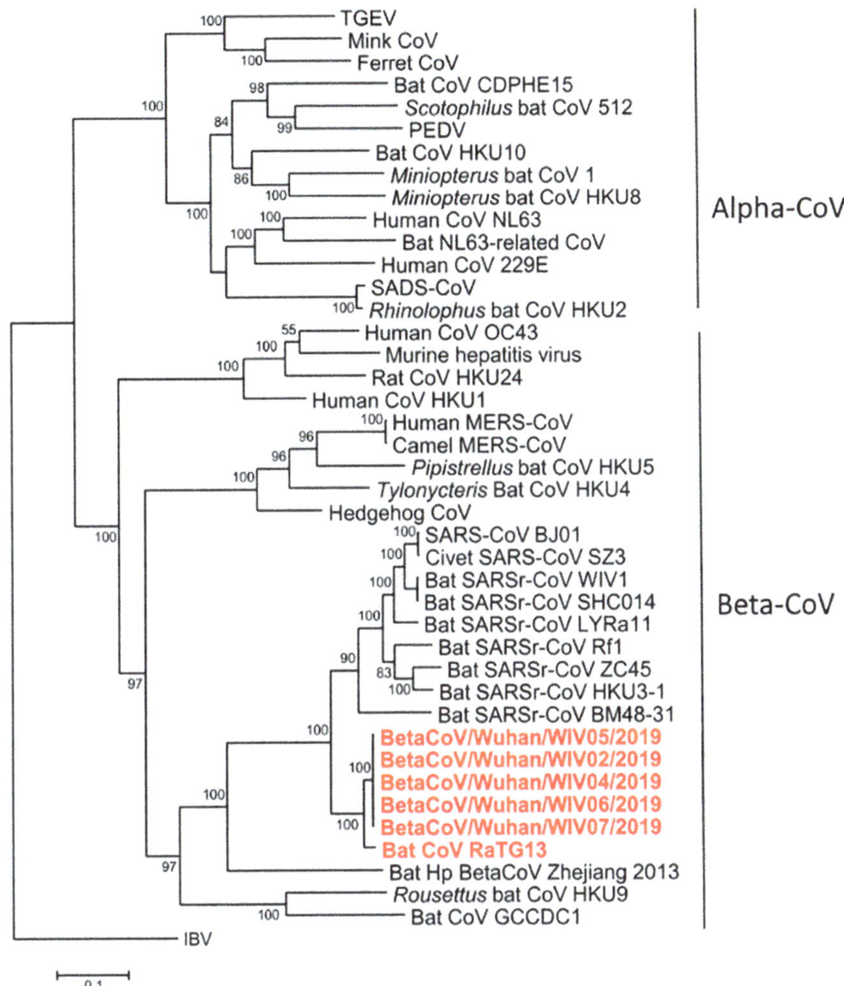

Figure 2-1. Sequence similarities based on the whole-genome sequence of SARS-CoV-2

SARS-CoV, the amino acid sequences of the seven conserved replicase domains in *open reading frame 1ab* (*ORF1ab*) — used for species classification—are 94.4% identical between SARS-CoV-2 and SARS-CoV. This suggests that the two viruses originated from the same species. Figure 2-1 shows the tree based on the whole-genome sequence similarities across SARS-CoV-2 and other coronaviruses.

2.1.2 *Animal host*

Growing evidence suggests that bats, notably Chinese horseshoe bats, are natural reservoirs of a large number of coronavirus species. According to a serological study on the rural residents living close to the natural habitat of cave-dwelling bats, 2.7% was found to be sero-positive for bat coronaviruses, suggesting a potentially common exposure of humans to coronaviruses in bats. Nonetheless, most species of bats inhabit tropical and subtropical rainforests or caves far from areas of human activities. Therefore, viruses derived from bats often need to evolve in some semi-domestic mammals (intermediate hosts) to eventually spread to humans after undergoing specific mutations and recombination. It is now believed that the initial host of SARS-CoV-2 is the Chinese horseshoe bat, whose subspecies are widely distributed in Southern China, Asia, the Middle East, Africa, and Europe. The latest study shows that pangolins are suspected as a potential animal host of SARS-CoV-2. The genome sequence of the β coronavirus isolated from pangolins was 99% identical to those in infected people in the protein sequence of the receptor-binding domain (RBD). However, multiple intermediate hosts could exist, and further studies are needed to identify them. The discovery of these animal hosts is of great significance for the prevention and control of the source of SARS-CoV-2.

2.1.3 *Types of transmission sources*

At present, the major source of transmission is the patients infected with SARS-CoV-2. Asymptomatic transmission seems to be possible, which was uncommon in the SARS epidemic. It is difficult to diagnose and isolate such carriers, who do not show symptoms. This makes it easy for sources of transmission to grow in communities, increasing the difficulty of controlling the spread of the disease. Some studies also suggest that patients could be infectious during the incubation period. Additionally, SARS-CoV-2 has been detected in convalescent patients, suggesting that they, too, could be infectious.

2.1.4 *Mutations in the virus*

As of end February 2020, whole-genome sequences of SARS-CoV-2 in different samples have been nearly identical without noticeable mutations. Results from the close surveillance of SARS-CoV-2 also suggested an absence of noticeable mutations, regardless of whether the virus was isolated from the environment, patients were in early stages of the outbreak, or samples were recent. Huashan Hospital affiliated to Fudan University published that the genome sequences of the virus isolated from imported cases in Shanghai shared more than 99% sequence homology with initial isolates in Wuhan. Whole-genome sequencing analysis by the World Health Organization (WHO) of 104 strains of the SARS-CoV-2 virus, isolated from patients in different localities with symptom onset, showed 99.9% homology without noticeable mutation.

However, based on knowledge about the coronaviruses, SARS-CoV-2 is a positive-sense single-stranded RNA virus. This group of viruses is prone to mutation and recombination, which can either increase or decrease its virulence.

2.2 Routes of Transmission

It is currently thought that the main routes of transmission are from person to person. Respiratory droplets produced when an infected person coughs, sneezes, and talks, make up the main mode of transmission, while close contact is another. Aerosol transmission is also possible under special conditions. Since SARS-CoV-2 strains were detected in samples of infected patients' feces in multiple locations, there is considerable risk that the virus can spread through the fecal-oral route. Further studies are needed to examine the existence of mother-to-child transmission.

2.2.1 *Respiratory droplet transmission*

Respiratory droplets remain the key route for SARS-CoV-2 transmission. Susceptible people can get infected after inhaling droplets released when an infected person coughs, sneezes, or talks.

2.2.2 *Transmission by indirect contact*

SARS-CoV-2 can also spread via indirect contact with infected individuals. Droplets containing coronavirus are deposited on surfaces, and susceptible people can be infected after their hands touched these surfaces before further touching their oral, nasal and other mucous membranes. When authorities in Guangdong, Shandong, and other provinces examined the residences of diagnosed patients, they detected SARS-CoV-2 on the surfaces of objects such as door knobs and smartphones. In theory, there is a possibility that SARS-CoV-2 could infect the respiratory tract through the conjunctiva, but recent clinical data of 67 confirmed or suspected cases of COVID-19 did not support this channel of transmission. Further studies are needed to investigate this route.

2.2.3 *Fecal-oral transmission*

More evidence is needed to confirm fecal-oral transmission. SARS-CoV-2 was detected in stool specimens of infected patients in Wuhan, Shenzhen, and even the United States, suggesting that the virus can proliferate and stay in the digestive tract. These results indicate a possibility of fecal-oral transmission, but it is not clear whether eating food contaminated by the virus can result in new infections. Additionally, others proposed that the virus in feces may be redistributed in droplets by forming aerosols, which too calls for further investigation.

2.2.4 *Aerosol transmission*

Aerosol transmission occurs when droplet nuclei, composed of proteins and pathogens left behind after droplets in the air dry up, float through distances in the form of aerosols. The aerosol transmission of SARS-CoV-2 may be possible if one is exposed to a high level of aerosols in an enclosed area for an extended period of time. However, no explicit evidence confirms that SARS-CoV-2 can transmit through aerosols.

2.2.5 *Mother-to-child transmission*

It was reported that the throat swab of a neonate born to a woman with COVID-19 tested positive for SARS-CoV-2 30 hours after birth, suggesting the possibility of mother-to-child transmission. However, a retrospective study analyzed nine cases and showed that the virus would not be passed on to the fetus during the last trimester of infected women. Neither was there evidence for intrauterine infection caused by vertical transmission. Nonetheless, transmission through physical contact between the mother and newborn cannot be ruled out. These findings are in accordance with what was observed in the SARS outbreak: no evidence of perinatal vertical transmission was found in newborns with mothers who developed SARS during pregnancy. The latest study finds that the receptor of SARS-CoV-2, angiotensin converting enzyme 2 (ACE2), is expressed at very low levels in all types of cells on the maternal-fetal interface, indicating an extremely small pool of potentially susceptible cell subpopulation to SARS-CoV-2 on the maternal-fetal interface. This may be the evidence that SARS-CoV-2 is unlikely to be vertically transmitted from mother to fetus. Of course, these conclusions still need to be verified by future studies.

After their field visits in China, WHO concluded that COVID-19 is mainly transmitted via droplets and close contact. In addition, the fecal-oral route and aerosol route in a relatively enclosed and narrow environment could transmit COVID-19; their roles and significance for COVID-19 transmission remain to be determined.

2.3 Susceptible Population

Everyone is susceptible to COVID-19 because the population has no immunity against this emerging infectious disease.

2.3.1 *Universal susceptibility*

Based on the age distribution of patients in China, people of all age groups are susceptible to SARS-CoV-2. People can be infected as long as the conditions for transmission are met. The analysis of 4,021 confirmed cases in China (diagnosis date as of January 26) also showed that people of all age groups are generally susceptible. Among these cases, 71.45% were 30 to 65 years old, and 0.35% were children under 10 years old. The risk of virus infection could increase in the elderly and people with underlying diseases such as asthma, diabetes, and cardiovascular disease. In another study, as of February 11, the majority of the 44,672 confirmed cases had been 30 to 70 years old (86.6%). Among all the cases, 44.1% and 35.1% were people older than 60 in Wuhan and the whole country, respectively.

2.3.2 *High-risk population*

The close contacts of COVID-19 patients and asymptomatic carriers are at high risk from SARS-CoV-2 infection. In particular, the health-care professionals and family members of the patient have very high risks of infection because they have frequent close contacts with the patient while treating, caring for, or visiting them. Among 138 hospitalized patients at Wuhan University Zhongnan Hospital, 29% were healthcare professionals. An analysis of 44,672 confirmed cases of COVID-19 (diagnosis date as of February 11) found that in the 422 medical facilities treating COVID-19 patients, 3,019 health workers were infected, making up 3.84% of the total confirmed cases.

2.4 Transmission Dynamics

The basic reproduction number (R_0, pronounced "R-naught") is used to reflect the transmission potential and the severity of an epidemic. It is the average number of secondary infections produced by a typical case of infection in a population where everyone is susceptible and no deliberate intervention is made. It is also an important parameter to describe the early stages of an infection. Simply put, R_0 describes how many people an infected person can infect. The larger the R_0, the more infectious the disease is. When the interpersonal virus transmission can be substantially and consistently curbed ($R_0 < 1$), it becomes feasible to control the spread and eradicate the disease.

The infectivity of a disease is not necessarily consistent with that perceived by the public. The infamous Ebola that causes hemorrhagic fever, and SARS, are far less infectious than mumps and measles. On the other hand, the risk of an infection is evaluated not only by R_0 but also by severity, fatality rate, and other factors.

In the early stages of COVID-19 outbreak (as of January 22), a retrospective study on 425 patients with COVID-19 showed that the mean incubation period was 5.2 days (95% confidence interval [CI], 4.1 – 7.0). The doubling time was 7.4 days, meaning the number of the infected doubled every 7.4 days, with a mean serial interval (the time between successive cases in a chain of transmission) of 7.5 days (95% CI: 5.3 – 19). The R_0 was estimated to be 2.2 (95% CI: 1.4 – 3.9), that is, every patient infected 2.2 people on average. According to another retrospective analysis on 265 patients in Shanghai conducted by a team from Huashan Hospital affiliated to Fudan University, the incubation period was 6.4 days (95% CI: 5.3 – 7.6) and the mean onset-admission interval was 5.5 days (95% CI: 5.1 – 5.9).

In the same period, many international epidemiology teams carried out studies on transmission dynamics. Their multiple efforts estimated the R_0 of COVID-19 to be 2.2 – 4.0 (a few estimated up to 6.0 – 7.0), and the doubling time to be 6.4 – 7.5 days, suggesting that interpersonal transmissibility of COVID-19 could be higher than that of SARS. In fact, there are differences in the mode of transmission between COVID-19 and SARS. From November 2002 when the first case of SARS was found to early February 2003, 305 cases were reported, far less than the number of SARS-CoV-2 infections. One important reason behind this huge margin is that SARS patients are not infectious during the incubation period. Despite the existence of super spreaders, its early transmission was far slower than that of COVID-19.

Typically, with the implementation of prevention and control measures, the R_0 would change. Therefore, in epidemiology, the factual R_0 is called the effective reproduction number (R_e). A study showed that the R_0 of COVID-19 in early stages was as large as 4.71 (4.50 – 4.92), but its effective reproduction number (R_e) dropped to 2.08 (1.99 – 2.18) as of January 22, 2020.

After comprehensive field visits in February 2020 in China, WHO concluded that COVID-19 differed from SARS in etiology. Its transmissibility is higher than that of SARS with a R_0 of 2.0–2.5.

References

1. Special Expert Group for Control of the Epidemic of Novel Coronavirus Pneumonia of the Chinese Preventive Medicine. An update on the epidemiological characteristics of novel coronavirus pneumonia (COVID-19). *Chinese Journal of Epidemiology.* 2020; 41(2):139–144.

2. Epidemiology Working Group for NCIP Epidemic Response. The epidemiological characteristics of an outbreak of 2019 novel coronavirus diseases (COVID-19) in China. *Chinese Journal of Epidemiology.* 2020;41(2):145–151.

3. Wuhan Municipal Health Commission. Wuhan Municipal Health Commission's Briefing on Current Outbreak of Pneumonia in Wuhan. [Internet]. 2019 [cited 2020 Feb 23]. http://wjw.wuhan.gov.cn/front/web/showDetail/2019123108989.2.

4. Chan JF, Yuan S, Kok KH, *et al.* A familial cluster of pneumonia associated with the 2019 novel coronavirus indicating person-to-person transmission: a study of a family cluster. *Lancet.* 2020;395(10223): 514–523.

5. Chen HJ, Guo JJ, Wang C, *et al.* Clinical characteristics and intrauterine vertical transmission potential of COVID-19 infection in nine pregnant women: a retrospective review of medical records. *Lancet.* 2020;395(10226):809–815.

6. Chen N, Zhou M, Dong X, *et al.* Epidemiological and clinical characteristics of 99 cases of 2019 novel coronavirus pneumonia in Wuhan, China: a descriptive study. *Lancet.* 2020;395(10223):507–513.

7. Li H, Mendelsohn E, Zong C, *et al.* Human-animal interactions and bat coronavirus spillover potential among rural residents in Southern China. *Biosafety Health.* 2019;1(2):84–90.

8. Shen M, Peng Z, Xiao Y, *et al.* Modelling the epidemic trend of the 2019 novel coronavirus outbreak in China [Internet]. *bioRxiv.* 2020 [cited 2020 Jan 23]. https://www.biorxiv.org/content/10.1101/2020.01.23.916726v1.

9. Wang N, Li SY, Yang XL, *et al.* Serological Evidence of Bat SARS-Related Coronavirus Infection in Humans, China. *Virologica Sinica.* 2018;33(1):104–107.

10. World Health Organization. Statement on the second meeting of the International Health Regulations (2005) Emergency Committee regarding the outbreak of novel coronavirus (2019-nCoV) [Internet]. 2020 [cited 2020 Feb 23]. https://www.who.int/news-room/detail/30-

01-2020-statement-on-the-second-meeting-of-the-international-health-regulations-(2005)-emergency-committee-regarding-the-outbreak-of-novel-coronavirus-(2019-ncov).

11. Zheng QL, Duan T, Jin LP. Single-Cell RNA Expression Profiling of ACE2 and AXL in the Human Maternal–Fetal Interface. *Reproductive and Developmental Medicine* [Internet]. 2020 [cited 2020 Feb 23]. http://www.repdevmed.org/preprintarticle.asp?id=278679.

12. Zhou P, Yang XL, Wang XG, *et al.* A pneumonia outbreak associated with a new coronavirus of probable bat origin. *Nature.* 2020;579: 270–273.

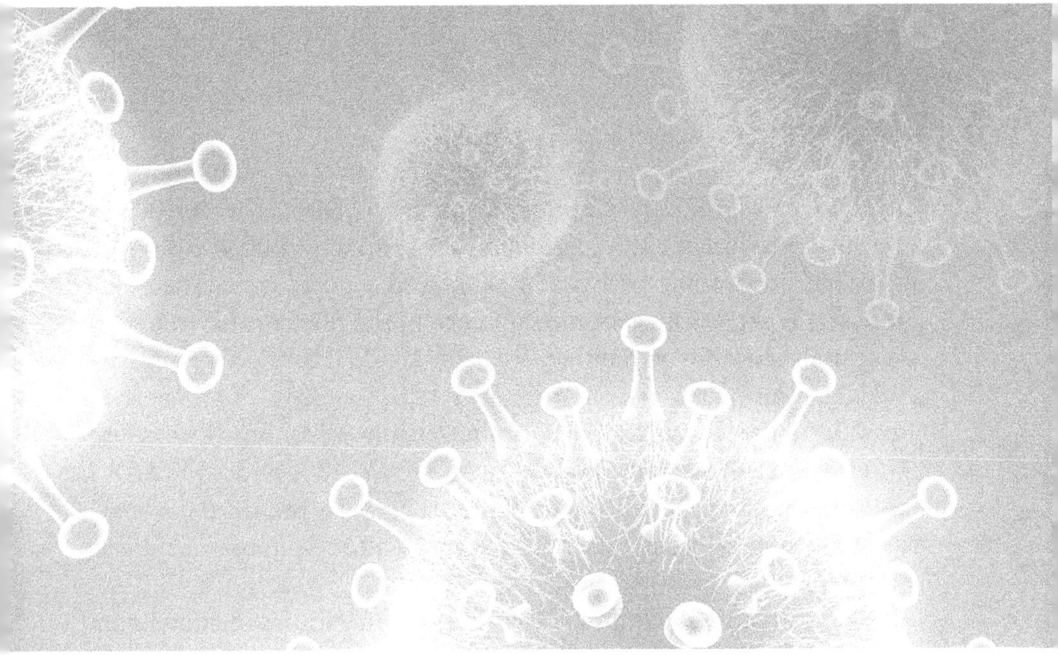

Part 2

Etiology and Pathogenesis

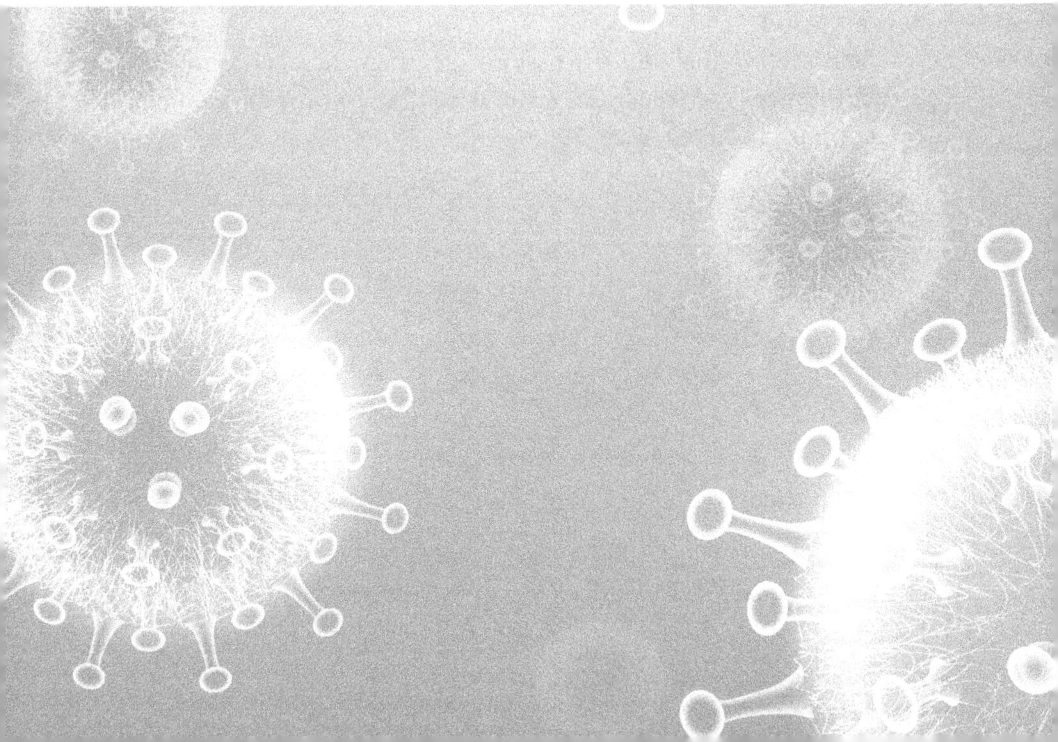

On January 7, 2020, Chinese Center for Disease Control and Prevention (China CDC) identified the pathogen isolated from multiple viral pneumonia patients in Wuhan as a novel coronavirus. On January 11, the whole genome sequence of the first coronavirus strain was published and on January 12, the World Health Organization (WHO) temporarily named the virus "2019-nCoV". On February 11, 2020, the International Committee on Taxonomy of Viruses (ICTV) officially named the virus "SARS-CoV-2". Besides the SARS-CoV in 2003 and the MERS-CoV in 2012, this is the third coronavirus in the past 20 years that causes severe acute respiratory syndrome in humans.

Coronaviruses constitute a large virus family found in animals and humans. It was first discovered in 1968 and was officially named by ICTV as the family of *Coronaviridae* in 1975. Coronaviruses are positive-sense single-stranded RNA viruses with genome sizes of 26–32 kb and have the largest genomes among RNA viruses. Coronaviruses have been isolated and identified in a variety of bird hosts and mammals, including vertebrates like camels, bats, mice, rats, dogs, and cattle. Currently, pathogenic coronaviruses in the human population include SARS-CoV, MERS-CoV, HCoV-HKU1, HCoV-NL63, HCoV-OC43, HCoV-229E, and the emerging SARS-CoV-2.

This section includes discussions of systematics, morphology and structure, genome structure, natural origin, and mechanisms of cell infection of SARS-CoV-2.

Chapter 3
Morphology, Systematics, and Structure

3.1 Position in Systematics

From a systematic perspective, coronaviruses belong to the *Coronavirus* genus, in the subfamily *Orthocoronavirinae*, family *Coronaviridae*, and order Nidovirales.

There are four *Coronavirus* genera, namely *Alpha-*, *Beta-*, *Gamma-* and *Deltacoronavirus*. In 2018, the ICTV divided the genus *Betacoronavirus* further into five subgenera, namely *Embecovirus*, *Sarbecovirus*, *Merbecovirus*, *Nobecovirus*, and *Hibecovirus* (Table 3-1). The first four subgenera correspond to the original A, B, C, and D evolutionary lineages in the genus *Betacoronavirus*. The viruses in subgenus *Hibecovirus* were isolated from bats in China and evolved from *Betacoronaviruses*, which are closely related phylogenetically to those in subgenus *Sarbecovirus*. The mammal-infecting coronaviruses mostly come from the genera *Alpha-* and *Betacoronavirus*, while those that infect birds mostly come from the genera of *Gamma-* and *Deltacoronavirus*. SARS-CoV-2 is currently classified under the subgenus of *Sarbecovirus* in the genus of *Betacoronavirus*.

The first strain of human coronavirus was isolated in 1965. The virion presents obvious club-shaped particle protrusions on its outer membrane when observed under an electron microscope (EM),

Table 3-1. Subgenera of *Betacoronavirus* genus and common viral species

Subgenus of *Betacoronavirus*	Common viral species
Embecovirus	*Human coronavirus HKU1* *Human coronavirus OC43* *Murine coronavirus*
Sarbecovirus	*SARS-CoV*
Merbecovirus	*MERS-CoV* *Tylonycteris bat coronavirus HKU4* *Pipistrellus bat coronavirus HKU5*
Nobecovirus	*Rousettus bat coronavirus HKU9*
Hibecovirus (new subgenus added in 2018)	*Bat Hp-betacoronavirus Zhejiang2013*

which resembles the crowns of medieval European emperors. The virus was hence named "coronavirus", derived from the Latin word *corona*, meaning "crown".

The morphology of SARS-CoV-2 resembles that of other coronaviruses. The viral particle is enveloped by a lipid bilayer with three glycoproteins on its surface: spike (S), envelope (E), and membrane (M) proteins. The viral particles are irregularly shaped with an average diameter of 100 nm (ranging from 60–220 nm). They are pleomorphically shaped and often seem spherical or oval.

On January 24, 2020, China CDC published the EM picture of the first successfully isolated SARS-CoV-2 strain, as shown in Figure 3-1 (SARS-CoV-2 indicated by arrows). Multiple typical irregular particulate protrusions can be seen surrounding the virus. On February 11, the US National Institute of Allergy and Infectious Diseases (NIAID) acquired images of SARS-CoV-2 with scanning and transmission electron microscopy (Figure 3-2). In this image, the ultra-microstructures are revealed and match the typical morphology of coronaviruses, such as the internal nucleocapsid structure and the spike protrusions on the surface of the viral particles. In the ultra-thin section of human airway epithelium, free viral particles are

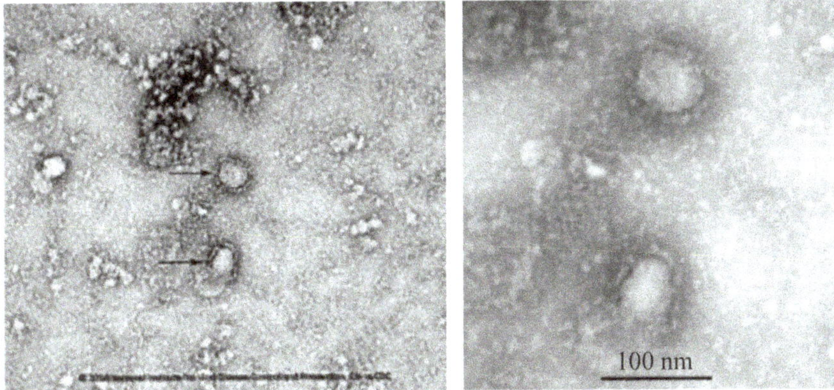

Figure 3-1. Electron microscopy images of SARS-CoV-2. Arrows indicate the isolated virus particles (cited from the official website of China CDC)

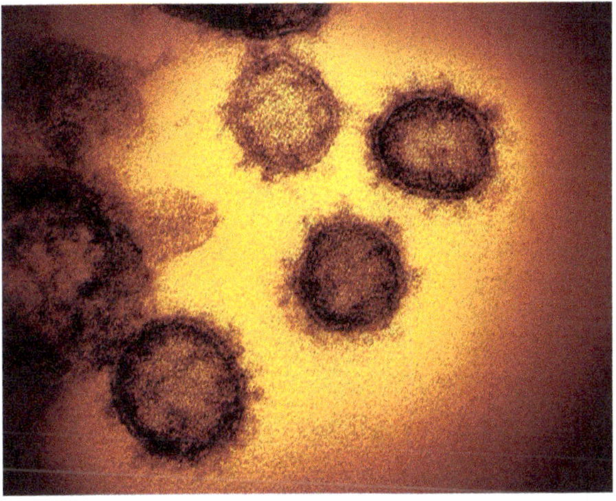

Figure 3-2. Colorized electron microscopy images of SARS-CoV-2 (cited from the official website of US NIAID)

observed outside the cells, while virus components can be seen within the cytoplasmic inclusion bodies bound to the membrane (Figure 3-3).

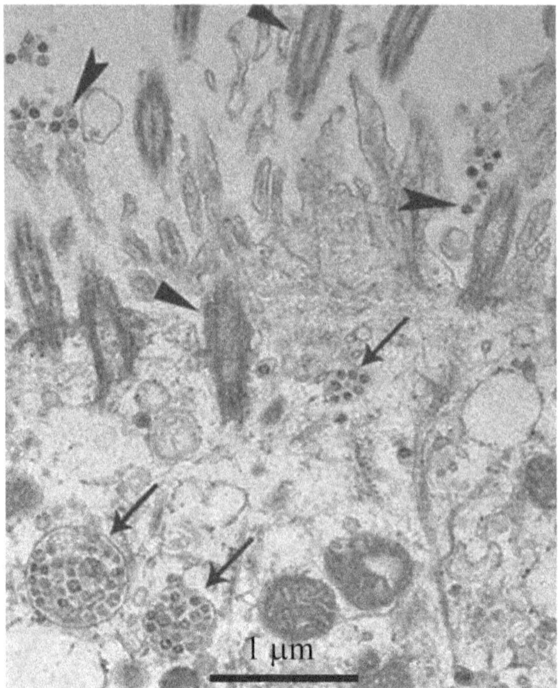

Figure 3-3. Transmission electron microscope image of SARS-CoV-2 particles in the ultra-thin section of human airway epithelium. Triangles point out airway epithelial cell cilia, arrowheads indicate extracellular virions, and arrows point out the inclusion bodies (Zhu N, Zhang D, Wang W, *et al.* A novel coronavirus from patients with pneumonia in China. *N Engl J Med.* 2020;382(8):727–733.)

3.2 Evolutionary Analyses of the Genome

As of February 23, 2020, there are more than 200 genomes of SARS-CoV-2 uploaded onto shared platforms such as GenBank, GISAID, and Genome Warehouse. Because coronaviruses have an extensive range of hosts and unique structural characteristics in the genomes, they are highly prone to genetic recombination during evolution and are genetically diverse. This section will navigate the comparative genomics and evolutionary analyses based on comparisons of the whole-genome sequences, single genes, and protein sequences.

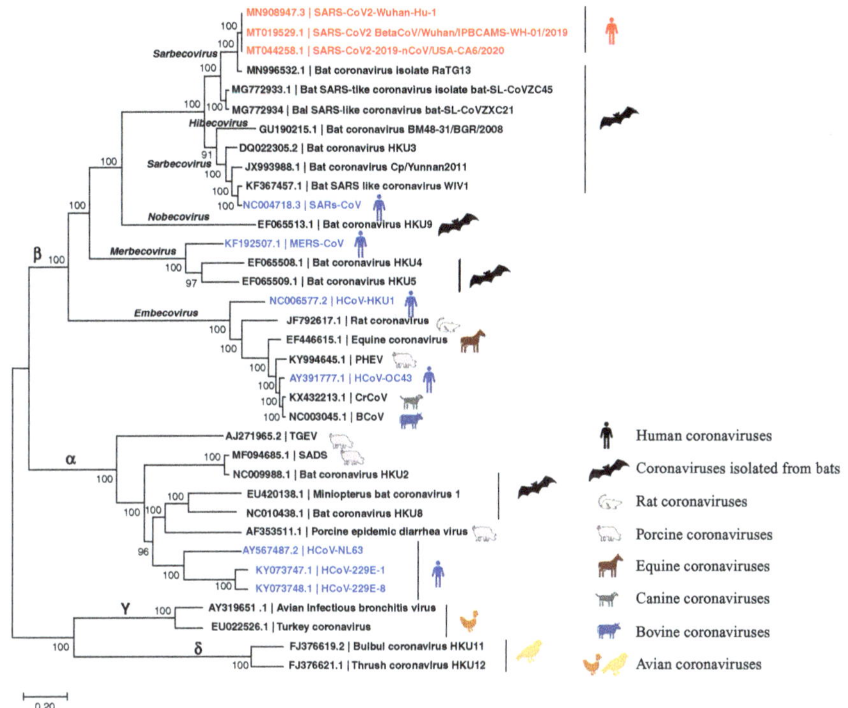

Figure 3-4.   Phylogenetic tree based on whole-genome sequences

3.2.1 *Evolutionary analysis based on whole viral genomes*

Based on the comparisons of whole genomes, Figure 3-4 shows the results of a phylogenetic analysis of SARS-CoV-2, together with representative coronaviral genomes downloaded from the US National Center of Biotechnology Information. The coronaviruses are distinctively classified into four genera, i.e. *Alpha-*, *Beta-*, *Gamma-* and *Deltacoronavirus*. As shown in this phylogenetic tree, the upper clades of the alpha and beta genera of coronaviruses infect humans, as well as mammals such as bats, horses, pigs, cattle, and dogs. The coronaviruses that infect birds are mainly derived from the gamma and delta genera, which are located in the lower clades of the phylogenetic tree.

SARS-CoV-2 belongs to the same coronavirus lineages as MERS-CoV and SARS-CoV. The *Sarbecovirus* subtypes in the *Betacoronavirus* subgenus can be further split into three phylogenetic clades. The first clade includes the clinically isolated SARS-CoV-2 strains and the bat coronavirus RaTG13 (Bat-CoV-RaTG13, GenBank Accession MN996532.1). The second clade is composed of two SARS-like strains derived from bats in Zhoushan in eastern China (Bat-SL-CoV-ZC45, GenBank Accession MG772933.1 and Bat-SL-CoV-ZXC21, GenBank Accession MG772934.1). The third clade includes the human-infecting SARS-CoV and multiple SARS-like strains with similar viral genomes derived from bats in southwest China. Judging by the genetic distance, SARS-CoV-2 is closer to Bat-Cov-RaTG13 isolate and bat-derived SARS-like viral strains than to SARS-CoV.

Comparisons of nucleotide sequence similarity based on sequencing contigs show that the Bat-Cov-RaTG13 isolate is the closest neighbor to SARS-CoV-2 isolates from both China and the US. This strain of bat coronavirus was isolated from the bats in Yunnan province of China, with an identity of 96.2% in the nucleotide sequences. The next were two strains of bat coronaviruses Bat-SL-CoV-ZC45 and Bat-SL-CoV-ZXC21, with similarities of 88.1% and 88.0% respectively, and they had a similarity of 79.6% with the SARS-CoV genome (Table 3-2).

According to the phylogenetical analysis (Figure 3-4) and the evidence from genomic similarities, SARS-CoV-2 is a novel β-coronavirus that belongs to the *Sarbecovirus* subgenus in the genus of *Betacoronavirus*.

3.2.2   *Based on single genes in the viral genome*

Further sequence comparisons on single genes show significant differences in multiple regions between SARS-CoV-2 and SARS-CoV, including the S- and N-terminals of *ORF1a*, *ORF3*, *E*, *ORF6*, *ORF7*, *ORF8*, and the middle parts of *N*.

As shown in Table 3-2, the *S* gene of SARS-CoV-2 had a 73.4% similarity with that of SARS-CoV, and 93.1% with that of Bat-Cov-RaTG13. In comparisons with other structural genes *E*, *M*, and *N*, gene *E* has the highest similarity of more than 90%. The similarities of *M* and *N* genes of SARS-CoV-2 compared to SARS-CoV were 85.6% and 88.8% respectively.

Table 3-2. Nucleotide and amino acid sequence similarities of SARS-CoV-2 and its related sequences (nucleotide/amino acid, %)

Name of sequence	Whole genome	ORF1a	ORF1b	S	ORF3a	E	M	ORF6	ORF7a	ORF7b	ORF8	N
SARS-CoV BJ01	79.6	79.6/ 80.8	86.2/ 95.7	73.4/ 76.9	75.3/ 72.6	94.7/ 96.0	85.6/ 90.5	75.8/ 67.2	82.8/ 86.0	84.8/ 81.4	51.1/ —	88.8/ 91.2
SARS-CoV Tor2	79.6	79.6/ 80.9	86.2/ 95.8	73.4/ 76.7	75.4/ 72.6	94.7/ 96.0	85.6/ 90.5	76.3/ 68.9	82.8/ 86.0	84.8/ 81.4	51.1/ —	88.8/ 91.2
Bat-Cov- RaTG13	96.2	96.0/ 98.0	97.3/ 99.3	93.1/ 97.7	96.3/ 97.8	96.3/ 97.8	95.5/ 99.6	95.6/ 97.5	95.6/ 97.5	99.2/ 97.7	97.0/ 95.0	96.9/ 99.9
Bat-SL- CoV-ZC45	88.1	91.0/ 95.7	86.1/ 96.0	77.8/ 82.3	87.8/ 90.9	98.7/ 100.0	93.4/ 98.6	88.8/ 87.6	88.8/ 87.6	94.7/ 93.0	88.5/ 94.2	91.2/ 94.3
Bat-SL-CoV- ZXC21	88.0	90.9/ 95.7	86.2/ 95.8	77.1/ 81.7	88.9/ 92.0	98.7/ 100.0	93.4/ 98.6	89.1/ 88.4	89.1/ 88.4	95.5/ 93.0	88.5/ 94.2	91.2/ 94.3

When comparing SARS-CoV-2 to bat-derived Bat-SL-CoV-ZC45 and Bat-SL-CoV-ZXC21, the sequence identity in *ORF1b* (approximately 86%) was lower than that in *ORF1a* (approximately 90%). In other words, the *ORF1b* gene in SARS-CoV-2 is different than bat-derived coronaviruses, forming a unique clade. This indicates a possible recombination event in the *ORF1b* gene that is likely to have happened in bat-derived coronaviruses. Figures 3-5 to 3-8 show the respective phylogenetic trees based on

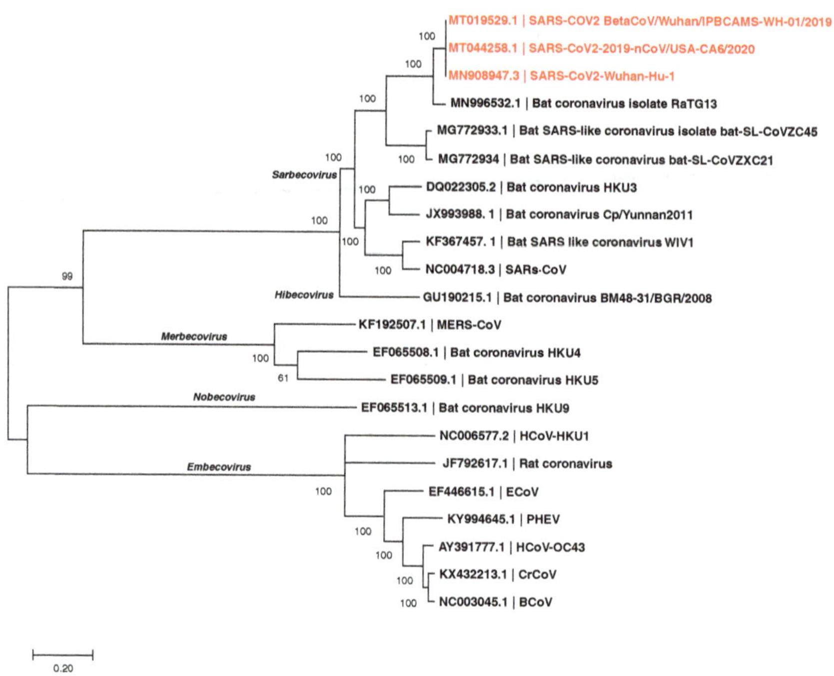

Figure 3-5.   Phylogenetic tree of the *S* genes in *β*-coronaviruses

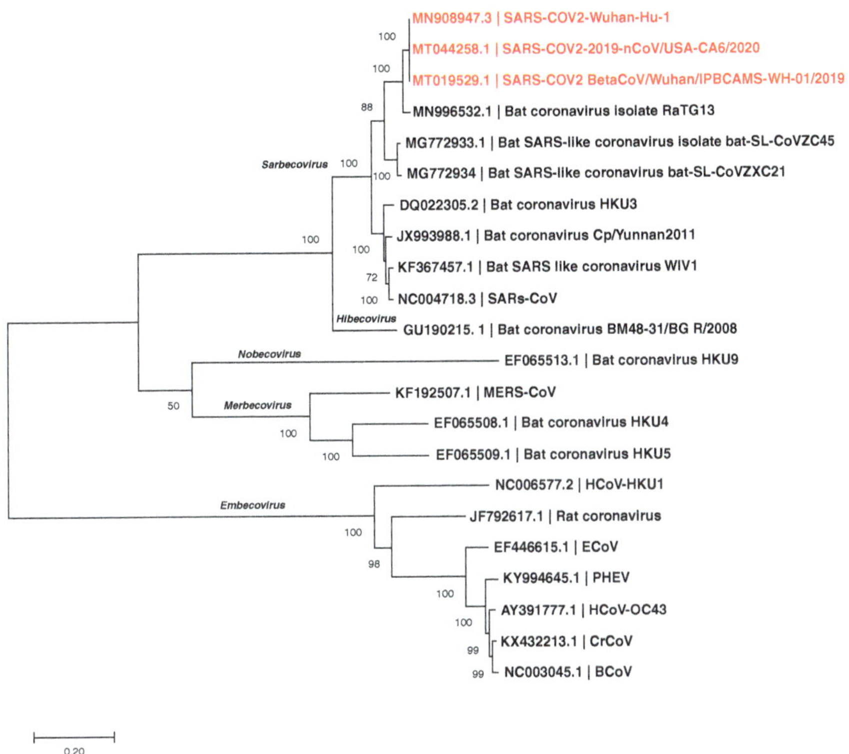

Figure 3-6. Phylogenetic tree of the N genes in β-coronaviruses

genes *S, N, ORF1a*, and *ORF1b*. As shown in Figures 3-7 and 3-8, in the aspect of evolutionary relationships, the *ORF1b* gene of SARS-CoV-2 was relatively farther from those of Bat-SL-CoV-ZC45 and Bat-SL-CoV-ZXC21, while SARS-CoV-2's *ORF1a* gene was closer to the two counterparts.

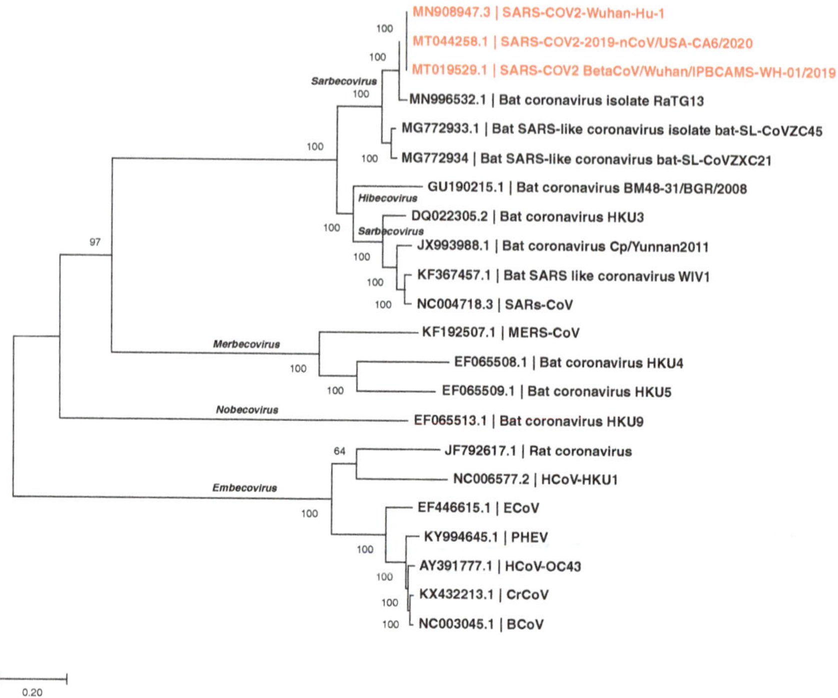

Figure 3-7.   Phylogenetic tree of the *ORF1a* genes in β-coronaviruses

3.2.3 *Comparative genomics analysis based on amino acid sequences*

SARS-CoV-2 and Bat-Cov-RaTG13 are highly identical in their protein sequences, with identities of 95.0–99.9% in amino acid sequences (Table 3-2). Despite the considerable similarity between SARS-CoV-2 and SARS-CoV, they showed significant differences in some coding genes. For example, the identity of *ORF8*-encoded protein with that of SARS-CoV is less than 40%, while the identity of *ORF3*-encoded protein

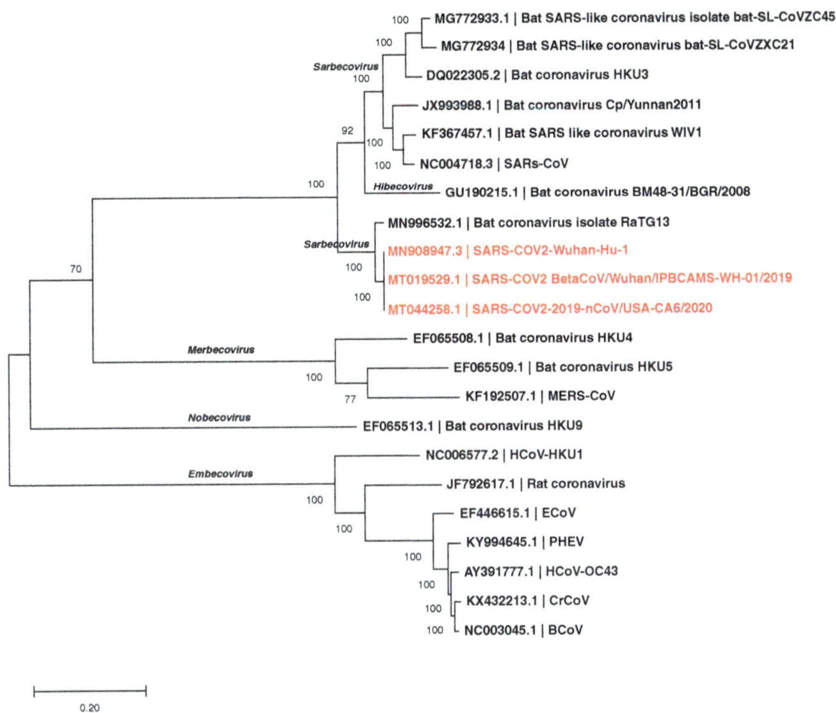

Figure 3-8.   Phylogenetic tree of the *ORF1b* genes in β-coronaviruses

is only 72.6%. However, *ORF8*-encoded proteins in Bat-SL-CoV-ZC45, Bat-SL-CoV-ZXC21, and Bat-Cov-RaTG13 are surprisingly similar to that in SARS-CoV-2, with amino acid sequence identities between 94% and 95%. Similarly, the *ORF1a*- and *ORF1b*-encoded proteins are highly conserved across SARS-CoV-2, Bat-SL-CoV-ZC45, and Bat-SL-CoV-ZXC21, with amino acid sequence identities between 95% and 96%, even though there were minor differences in the nucleotide sequences as mentioned above.

The most important protein in SARS-CoV-2, the S protein, showed 81.7% identity in amino acid sequences compared to that of Bat-SL-CoV-ZXC21, and is 76% similar to the S protein of SARS-CoV. Further analyses on the S1 and S2 subunits of the S protein suggest that in SARS-CoV-2, the S2 subunit is more conserved, with an amino acid sequence identity of 93% when compared to Bat-SL-CoV-ZC45 and Bat-SL-CoV-ZXC21. This percentage is substantially higher than 68%, the amino acid sequence identity of S1 subunit. Figures 3-9 to 3-12 show the phylogenetic trees based on proteins S and N, as well as *ORF1a*- and *ORF1b*-encoded proteins.

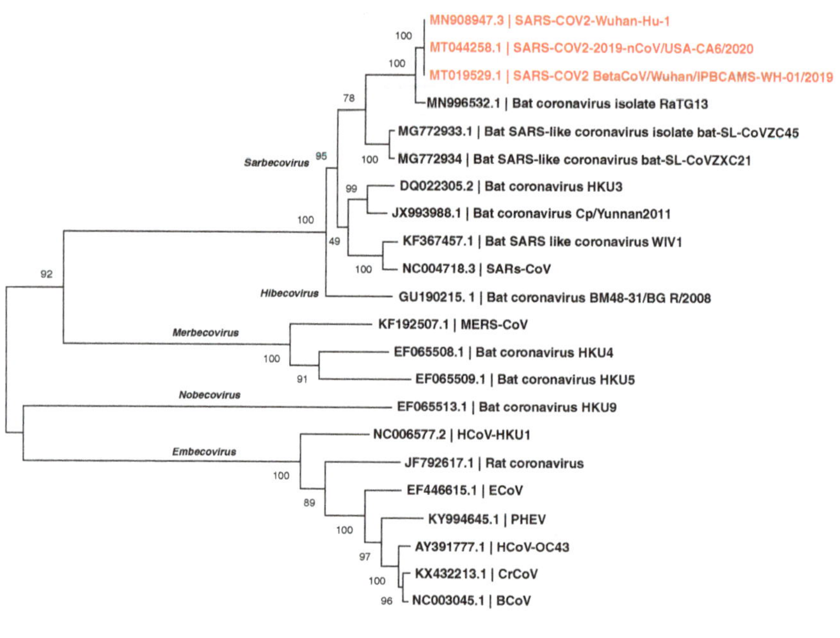

Figure 3-9.   Phylogenetic tree of the S proteins in β-coronaviruses

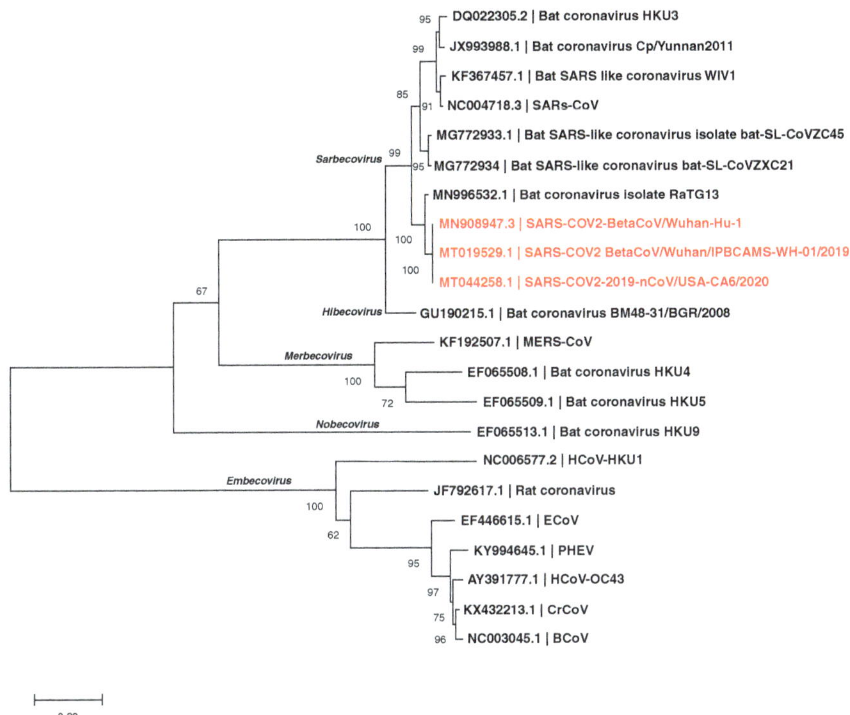

Figure 3-10. Phylogenetic tree of the N proteins in β-coronaviruses

As shown in Table 3-3, comparisons of amino acid sequence similarities of the 16 *ORF1ab*-encoded non-structural proteins (NSP) show no significant differences between SARS-CoV-2 and SARS-CoV.

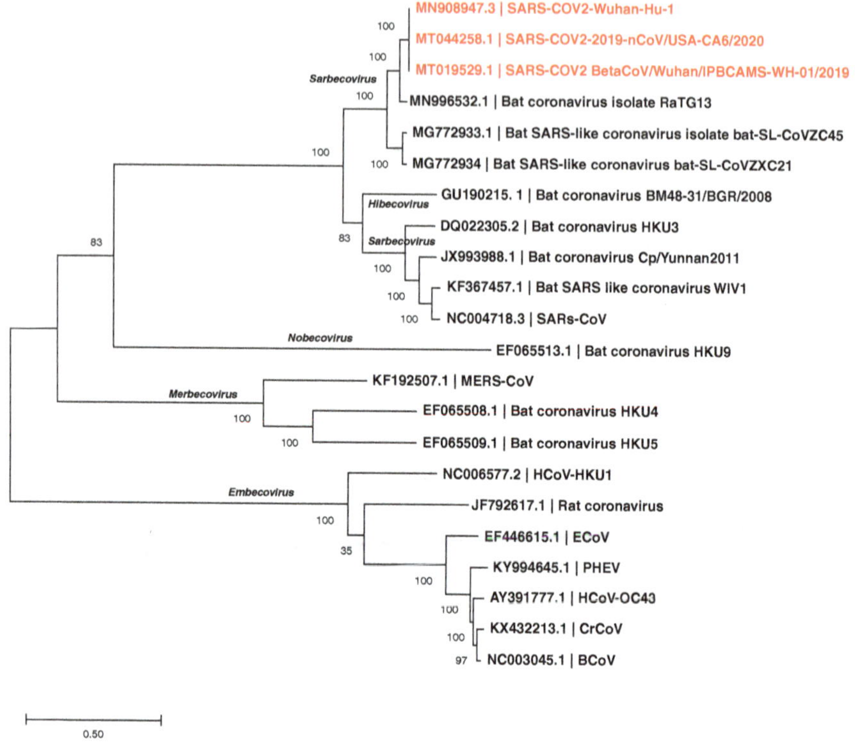

Figure 3-11.   Phylogenetic tree of the *ORF1a*-encoded proteins in β-coronaviruses

3.2.4 *Time series analysis*

As of February 10, 2020, according to the phylogenetic analysis of genomic data on Nextstrain (https://nextstrain.org/ncov), results based on a star-like tree model showed that the earliest appearance of SARS-CoV-2 was approximately mid-November 2019 (95% confidence interval of mid-October to early December, 2019).

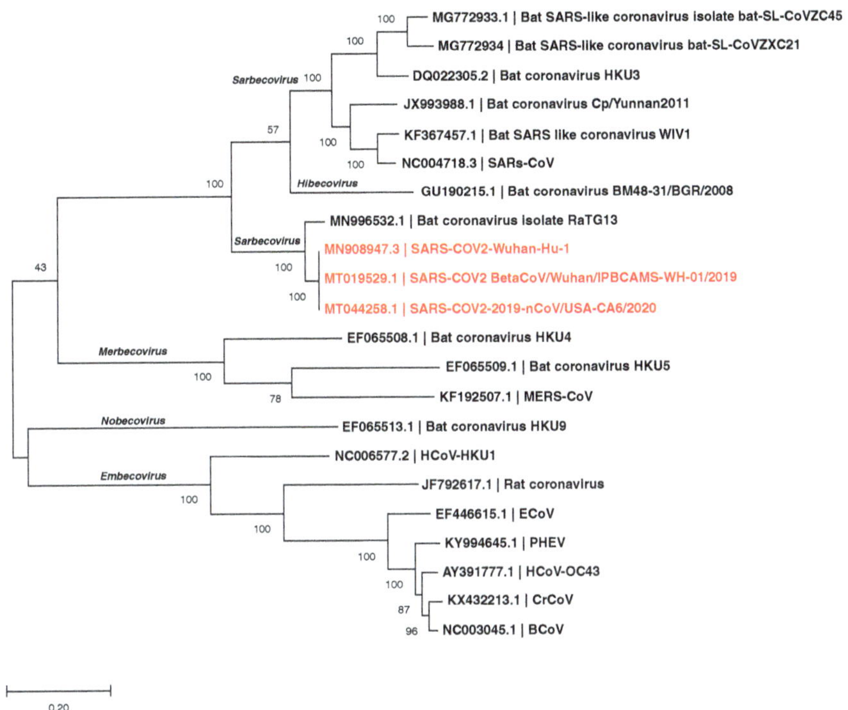

Figure 3-12.   Phylogenetic tree of the *ORF1b*-encoded proteins in β-coronaviruses

Table 3-3.   Amino acid sequence identities of NSP

	SARS-CoV-2 *vs.* Bat-SL-CoV-ZXC21 (%)	SARS-CoV-2 *vs.* SARS-CoV (%)
NSP1	96	84
NSP2	96	68
NSP3	93	76
NSP4	96	80
NSP5	99	96
NSP6	98	88
NSP7	99	99
NSP8	96	97
NSP9	96	97

(*Continued*)

Table 3-3.   (*Continued*)

	SARS-CoV-2 *vs.* Bat-SL-CoV-ZXC21 (%)	SARS-CoV-2 *vs.* SARS-CoV (%)
NSP10	98	97
NSP11	85	85
NSP12	96	96
NSP13	99	100
NSP14	95	95
NSP15	88	89
NSP16	98	93

3.3 Structure of the Viral Genome

SARS-CoV-2 is a positive-sense single-stranded RNA virus in the *Betacoronavirus* genus, *Orthocoronavirinae* subfamily, and the *Coronaviridae* family. The virus is enveloped with the E protein, with a genome size of approximately 29,891 nucleotides (nt).

Bioinformatic analyses of the nucleotide sequence homology and open reading frame (ORF) prediction among viruses in the *Betacoronavirus* genus suggest that SARS-CoV-2 has 12 potential ORFs (Figure 3-13), which are respectively 5'-replicase (ORF1ab)-structural proteins (Spike-Envelope-Membrane-Nucleocapsid)-3'.

The lengths of the 5'- and 3'-untranslated regions (UTR) are 265nt and 229nt, respectively. The 5'-UTR contains the ribosome binding site and the transcription initiation signal, while the 3'-UTR contains the transcription termination signal. These structures participate in messenger RNA transcription and protein translation. There are also multiple stem-loop structures in the two regions involved in the regulation of viral replication.

The gene *ORF1ab* encodes the replicase polyprotein (pp) 1a and pp1ab. Specific cleavages of the two proteins by NSP3 and NSP5 yield other NSPs in NSP1 – NSP16. Table 3-4 lists the functions of each NSP protein. NSP1 is a vital regulatory molecule in antagonizing innate immunity. According to previous reports, in SARS-CoV infection, NSP1 participates in regulation of the calcineurin-nuclear

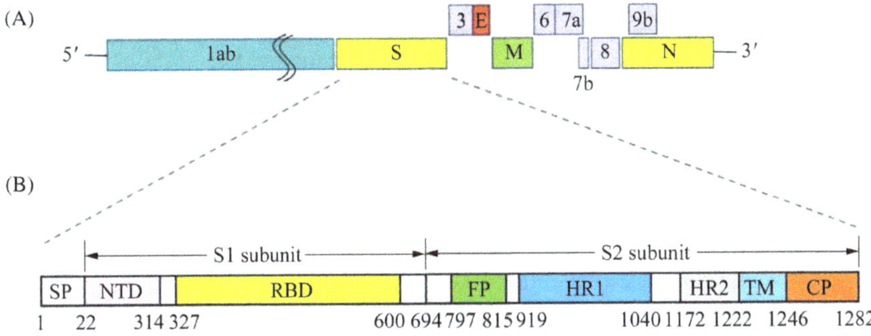

Figure 3-13.   Schematic illustration of the SARS-CoV-2 genome structure

A: potential ORFs in SARS-CoV-2 genome: *ORF1ab* encodes replicase polyprotein; *S, E, M,* and *N* encode the Spike protein, Envelope protein, Membrane protein, and Nucleocapsid protein respectively. **B**: structural domains in the S protein: SP, signal peptide; NTD, N'-terminal domain; RBD, receptor-binding domain; FP, fusion peptide; HR1 and HR2, heptad repeat 1 and 2; TM, transmembrane domain; CP, cytoplasmic domain. The start and end positions of the structural domains are annotated by the numbers in the figure. (Chan JF, Kok KH, Zhu Z, *et al.* Genomic characterization of the 2019 novel human-pathogenic coronavirus isolated from a patient with atypical pneumonia after visiting Wuhan. *Emerg Microbes Infect.* 2020;9(1):221–236.)

Table 3-4.   Biological functions and cleavage sites of NSP1 to 16

NSP	Predicted function / Function domain	Amino acid residue start/ end	Predicted cleavage site
NSP1	Inhibition of the host antiviral responses	M1 – G180	(LNGG'AYTR)
NSP2	Unknown	A181 – G818	(LKGG'APTK)
NSP3	Potential papain-like protease	A819 – G2763	(LKGG'KIVN)
NSP4	Forming complex with NSP3 and NSP6	K2764 – Q3263	(AVLQ'SGFR)
NSP5	Chymotrypsin-like protease	S3264 – Q3569	(VTFQ'SAVK)
NSP6	Forming complex with NSP3 and NSP4	S3570 – Q3859	(ATVQ'SKMS)
NSP7	Forming replicase complex with NSP8	S3860 – Q3942	(ATLQ'AIAS)
NSP8	Forming replicase complex with NSP7	A3943 – Q4140	(VKLQ'NNEL)

(Continued)

Table 3-4.   (*Continued*)

NSP	Predicted function / Function domain	Amino acid residue start/ end	Predicted cleavage site
NSP9	RNA/DNA binding activity	N4141 – Q4253	(VRLQ'AGNA)
NSP10	Forming replication fidelity complex with NSP14	A4254 – Q4392	(PMLQ'SADA)
NSP11	Short peptide at the end of ORF1a	S4393 – V4405	(to the end of ORF1a)
NSP12	RNA-dependent RNA polymerase	S4393 – Q5324	(TVLQ'AVGA)
NSP13	Helicase	A5325 – Q5925	(ATLQ'AENV)
NSP14	3'-5' exonuclease (ExoN)	A5926 – Q6452	(TRLQ'SLEN)
NSP15	Poly (U)-specific endoribonuclease (XendoU)	S6453 – Q6798	(PKLQ'SSQA)
NSP16	2'-O-ribose methyltransferase (2'-O-MT)	S6799 – N7096	(to the end of ORF1b)

Note: Apostrophe (') marks out the predicted enzymatic cleavage sites.

factors of activated T cell (CaN-NFAT) signaling pathway and promotes abnormal expressions of cytokines. The NSP12 and NSP13 are RNA-dependent RNA polymerase and helicase respectively, and are directly involved in viral replication. Thus, the cleavage activities of NSP3 and NSP5 have direct influence on subsequent viral replication levels. Since NSP5 is a virus-specific proteolytic enzyme, it is broadly considered to be a target for antiviral drugs. A recent study resolved its 3D structure with a resolution of 1.75 Å (1 Å = 0.1 nm) (Figure 3-14). NSP5 is a homodimer protein with three crucial structural domains, namely chymotrypsin- and picornavirus-3C protease-like domains I (residues 10–99), II (residues 100–182), and III (residues 198–303). Domain I and II both contain six-stranded antiparallel β-barrels that harbor the substrate-binding site between them. Domain III consists of five helical structures involved in the formation of the homodimer.

The *S* gene encodes the S protein, which comprises the S1 and S2 subunits. As shown in Figure 3-13, the S1 subunit consists of the N-terminal domain (NTD) and the receptor-binding domain (RBD).

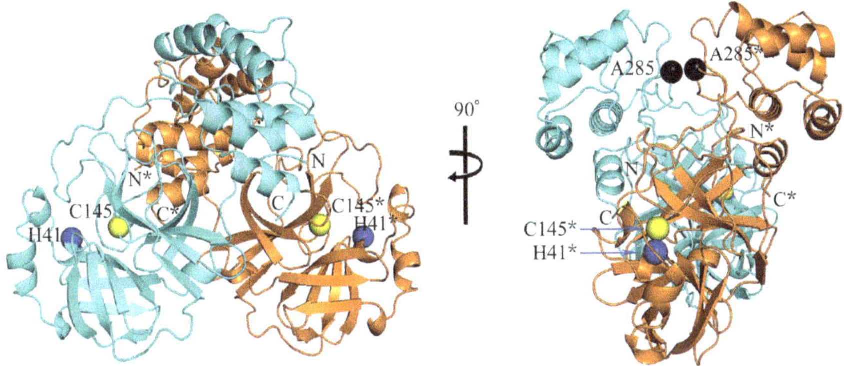

Figure 3-14.   Three-dimensional structure of NSP5

NSP5 is a homodimer protein, with the two monomers shown in blue and orange. N and C indicate the N-terminus and the C-terminus of the monomer in blue, while N* and C* indicate those of the monomer in orange. H41 and C145 represent histidine-41 and cysteine-145 respectively, which are both catalytic sites. A285 represents alanine-285, which is the location of domain III.
(Zhang LL, Lin DZ, Sun XY, *et al.* X-ray structure of main protease of the novel coronavirus SARS-CoV-2 enables design of α-ketoamide inhibitors. *bioRxiv.* (2020-02-17) [2020-02-23]. https://doi.org/10.1101/2020.02.17.952879.)

Both are crucial for the virus during the process of recognition and binding to the membrane receptors of the target cell. The S2 subunit consists of the fusion peptide (FP), the heptad repeat (HR) 1 and 2, the transmembrane domain (TM), and the cytoplasmic domain (CP), all with conserved amino acid sequences. When the S1 subunit binds with the membrane receptor angiotensin converting enzyme 2 (ACE2), composition of the S2 subunit changes. This in turn promotes the fusion of the viral envelope with the cellular or endosomal membrane of the target cell to release the viral RNA genome. The structure of the S protein and the virus entry mechanism will be substantiated in the next chapter.

The genes *ORF3*, *ORF6*, *ORF7a*, *ORF7b*, *ORF8*, and *ORF9b* encode the accessory proteins of the virus. Despite the unclear functions of these proteins in the life cycle of SARS-CoV-2, it was already reported in the literature that ORF3 and ORF6 inhibit the interferon (IFN) signaling pathway during infection to antagonize innate immunity. The ORF7 can upregulate the expression of interleukin 8 (IL8) and chemokine ligand 5 (CCL5) through the activation of nuclear factor kappa-B (NF-κB) signaling pathway. The ORF8 can provoke intracellular stress responses and promote the formation of NOD-like receptor family, pyrin domain-containing protein 3 (NLRP3) inflammasome. The functions of these proteins in SARS-CoV-2 need to be further investigated.

The *E*, *M*, and *N* genes encode the envelope, membrane, and nucleocapsid proteins, respectively. These proteins play important roles during the viral assembly, maturation, and shedding. The coronavirus has a relatively low E protein content. This protein is a trans-membrane structural protein that exhibits ion channel activity, with a molecular weight of 8 to 12 kilo-Dalton (kDa). Research has shown that E protein has no function in viral replication but its ion channel activity is one of the main causes of pathogenicity of coronaviruses. The M protein, whose content is the highest in the coronavirus, has a molecular weight of 25 to 30 kDa and three transmembrane structural domains. It serves a key role in maintaining the morphology of the virus. Research has shown that the M proteins form homodimers in the viral particle, which help in nucleocapsid binding and in maintaining the curvature of the viral envelope. The N protein is the only protein known in the nucleocapsid composition, and its N- and C-terminal domains (NTD and CTD) can bind to the coronavirus RNA. Research has shown that after high levels of phosphorylation, the N protein helps alter the structure of the nucleocapsid, which in turn specifically screens and binds to the coronavirus RNA.

Chapter 4
SARS-CoV-2 Natural Origins and Genomic Mutation

4.1 Origins of SARS-CoV-2

4.1.1 *Natural host*

Based on whole-genome sequence comparisons and phylogenetic analysis, SARS-CoV-2 is classified as a novel virus in the subgenus *Sarbecovirus* under the genus *Betacoronovirus*. Compared with the human-infecting SARS-CoV, the SARS-CoV-2 are closer related to the bat-derived SARS-like coronaviruses. Considering that both SARS-CoV and all aforementioned closely related viruses originated from bats, it is reasonable that SARS-CoV-2 also originated from bats. The intermediate host between bats and humans, however, cannot be determined so far.

Multiple pieces of evidence suggested the existence of intermediate hosts. Firstly, the emergence and epidemic spread of this virus was first reported in late December of 2019, during which the bat species living near Wuhan were still in hibernation. Secondly, in the Huanan Seafood Wholesale Market where wild animals were sold and the first cases were reported, no bats were being sold or displayed. Instead, the wet market featured non-aquatic animals such as porcupines, badgers, snakes, pangolins, and various birds. Furthermore, in the past SARS-CoV and MERS-CoV outbreaks, despite having bats as natural reservoirs, both viruses went through their intermediate host species before jumping to humans, the definitive hosts. For

SARS-CoV, the intermediate host is the civet cat; for MERS-CoV, the intermediate host is the dromedary camel. Therefore, SARS-CoV-2, the disease vector behind the COVID-19 outbreak in Wuhan, most likely started with bats as reservoir hosts, then mutated and evolved in their intermediate hosts, a yet unknown wild animal species, before eventually infecting humans.

In the previous chapter, we have established that the virus strain Bat-Cov-RaTG13 has the highest genetic similarity with SARS-CoV-2, with a whole-genome nucleotide similarity of 96.2% and a S protein amino acid similarity of 97.7%. This prompts us to investigate the possibility that SARS-CoV-2 directly evolved from Bat-CoV RaTG13.

Most of the amino acid differences between the two viruses are found in the receptor-binding domains (RBD), which determines the host specificity. One of the key proteins that mediate the virus to enter host cells, S protein, comprises subunits S1 and S2. The S1 subunit contains critical RBDs, although the S2 subunit, which constitutes the "stem" of the spike formed by S protein, is highly conserved across SARS-like coronaviruses. To infect host cells, the RBD must first bind with the surface protein on the host cell. For example, SARS-CoV binds with the ACE2 receptor expressed in the human airway epithelia and lung parenchyma. We will elaborate on this process in the next chapter. The S protein amino acid sequence in Bat-Cov-RaTG13 diverges from that in SARS-CoV-2 from position 435 to 510 (with a nucleotide and amino acid similarity of 75% and 78%, respectively). This region is the RBD motif responsible for the host specificity. Furthermore, out of the five critical amino acid residues in the RBD of Bat-Cov-RaTG13, only one is consistent with that of SARS-CoV-2 (Figure 4-1). Hence, it is unlikely that the virus jumped directly to humans from the bat. At least one intermediate host species is needed for this virus to mutate and recombine.

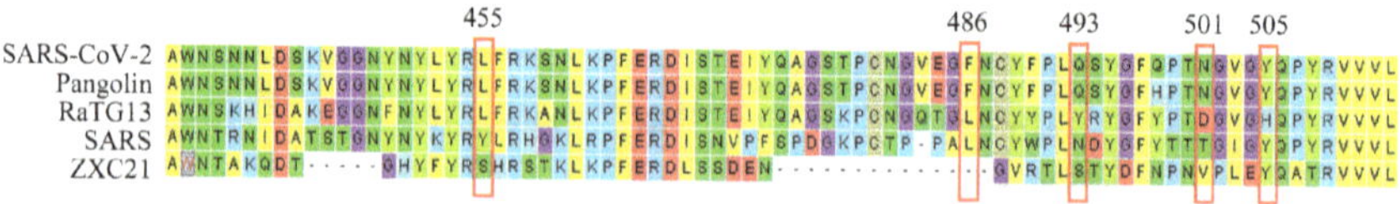

Figure 4-1.   Comparison of crucial amino acid sites of the S protein RBD

4.1.2 *Intermediate host*

Many research teams have analyzed the virome of pangolins and found that they carry viruses highly similar to SARS-CoV-2 in the genus *Betacoronavirus*. Their findings suggest that pangolins could be the intermediate host for SARS-CoV-2, which may have resulted from recombination between coronaviruses in pangolins and Bat-Cov-RaTG13.

So far, it is unclear whether SARS-CoV-2 has other intermediate forms after diverging from the pangolin coronavirus. On February 7, 2020, the research team from South China Agricultural University and Guangdong Laboratory for Lingnan Modern Agricultural Science and Technology announced in a news release that they found pangolins to be a potential intermediate host. Since then, multiple teams from China and other countries have discovered β-CoV in the viromes of Malayan pangolins (*Manis javanica*) that are similar to SARS-CoV-2. Although the genomes of these pangolin-derived coronaviruses were only 85.5–92.4% similar to that of SARS-CoV-2, lower than that of Bat-Cov-RaTG13, their S proteins have similarities as high as 90.4%, more than the 89.2% S protein similarity of Bat-Cov-RaTG13. In particular, their RBD motifs have only one amino acid change from that of SARS-CoV-2, and the five critical amino acid residues on the interface between ACE2 and their RBD are identical to that in SARS-CoV-2. Meanwhile, Bat-Cov-RaTG13 has only one out of these five amino acids identical to SARS-CoV-2 (Figure 4-1). Further protein interaction simulations also suggest that the S proteins in SARS-CoV-2 and the pangolin coronavirus can bind with the ACE2 in both humans and pangolins.

Further research implicated signs of possible recombination between pangolin coronavirus, Bat-Cov-RaTG13, and human SARS-CoV-2, but the evidence is not substantial. The similarity in the amino acid sequences of S1 subunit N-terminal domain (S1-NTD) is relatively low between the pangolin coronavirus and SARS-CoV-2, but their similarity increases around the region covering RBD and S2 (Figure 4-2). This suggests that recombination between Bat-Cov-RaTG13 and pangolin coronavirus may have occurred on a locus between S1-NTD and RBD regions. Nonetheless, despite the high

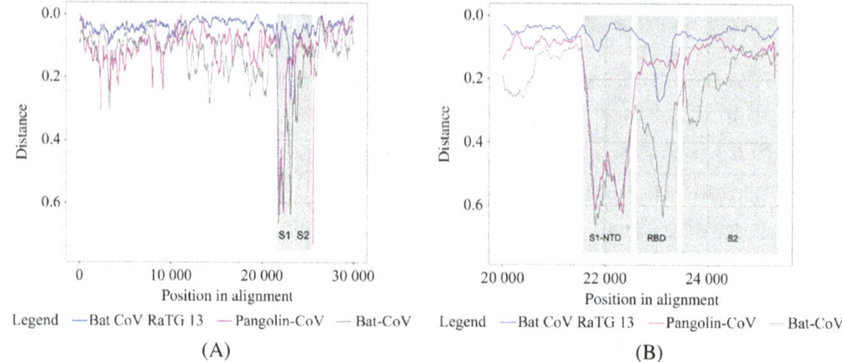

Figure 4-2. Genomic similarities between SARS-CoV-2 and bat- or pangolin-derived coronavirus A: comparison based on whole genomes; B: comparison of the S proteins. (Wong MC, Javornik Cregeen SJ, Ajami NJ, *et al.* Evidence of recombination in coronaviruses implicating pangolin origins of nCoV-2019. [J/OL]. *bioRxiv.* (2020-02-07) [2020-02-23]. https://doi.org/10.1101/2020.02.07.939207.)

amino acid similarity between the pangolin coronavirus and SARS-CoV-2, their nucleotide sequences are still relatively different. One possibility is that the recombination event was ancient, allowing for substantial genetic drift; another possibility is convergent evolution under selective pressure. Based on all existing evidence, however, neither hypothesis can be sufficiently supported. Still, although it is currently difficult to determine which scenario — convergent evolution, recombination, or both — drove the evolution of SARS-CoV-2, we must highlight the important role played by the intermediate host in this process. There could be more than one recombination event segregating Bat-Cov-RaTG13 and SARS-CoV-2, and pangolin may have only been involved in one of them.

Another difference between SARS-CoV-2 and pangolin coronavirus is at the junction of S1 and S2 subunits. To function properly, the two subunits S1 and S2 need to be cleaved by host protease. The cleavage site at the S1/S2 junction directly affects the efficiency of the cleavage and the infection, and is thus very critical. In SARS-CoV-2, new amino acid residues (-PRRA-) are inserted near the S1/S2 boundary. Together with the arginine (R) residue following this sequence, these residues form a cleavage site for the protease Furin. The insertion of this sequence is not observed in pangolin coronavirus and other bat coronaviruses but has been reported in the S protein in multiple coronaviruses, such as murine hepatitis virus JHM and human coronavirus HKU-1.

Another study proposed that snake could be an intermediate host based on sequence analyses and relative synonymous codon usage biases. Their hypothesis was later refuted due to the flaws in their study design.

4.2 Genomic Mutations

4.2.1 *Rate of evolution in SARS-CoV-2*

Based on the principles of molecular evolution, viruses are more likely to mutate faster when spreading in human populations. The mutant strains with higher transmissibility and favored by natural selection will spread more easily in the population. As a typical RNA virus, the average rate of evolution in coronaviruses is 10^{-4} nucleotide per site per year, and the viruses would mutate during every replication cycle. The mutation rates of SARS-CoV, MERS-CoV, avian influenza virus, and enterovirus are 0.8×10^{-3} to 2.4×10^{-3}, 8.76×10^{-4} to 1.37×10^{-3}, 1.8×10^{-3} to 8.4×10^{-3}, and 1.0×10^{-3} to 3.9×10^{-3} nucleotide substitution per site per year, respectively.

As of the end of February 2020, the sequences of SARS-CoV-2 isolated from different patients are 99.9% identical, suggesting a single source for this short period of time. However, clinically isolated strains from multiple places have already shown substantial heterogeneity. Researchers in Italy, Brazil, and the US analyzed the whole-genome data of 29 strains and found 15% of the loci are discordant. The time of sampling is highly correlated with the genetic distance between the viral strain and its ancestor strain. It is estimated that the most recent common ancestor (MRCA) dates back to November 25, 2019, and the rate of evolution is approximately 6.58×10^{-3} nucleotide per site per year, slightly higher than those of SARS-CoV and MERS-CoV.

4.2.2 *Types and proportions of mutations in SARS-CoV-2*

The SARS-CoV-2 database (2019nCoVR https://bigd.big.ac.cn/ncov,) hosted by China's National Genomics Data Center (NGDC) integrates SARS-CoV-2 data such as genomes and protein sequences publicly released by institutes such as Germany-based Global Initiative on Sharing All Influenza Data (GISAID), US National Center for Biotechnology Information (NCBI), China National GeneBank (CNGB), and China NGDC. As of February 20, 2020, the database encompasses a total of 179 genomes of clinically isolated SARS-CoV-2 strains. Using MN908947.3 as the reference sequence, the genomic similarities across these strains are all above 99.9%.

Among the 179 strains, 123 (68.7%) carry new mutations. There is a total of 188 single nucleotide polymorphisms (SNPs) and insertions or deletions (indels), among which 91 are non-synonymous mutations and 52 are synonymous mutations. The most prevalent missense mutations are ORF L85S, ORF3a G251V, ORF1ab L3606F, and ORF8 V62L, which are found in 36, 17, 10, and 6 strains, respectively. Another 3 strains carry premature translation termination codons, which are ORF1ab Y5124stop, ORF7a Q62stop, and S protein L861stop (Figure 4-3).

The Interactive Visualization of Phylogenomic data for SARS-CoV-2 (auspice, http://fight-ncov.genowis.com/ncov) performs big-data analyses on the viral genome sequences. By February 16,

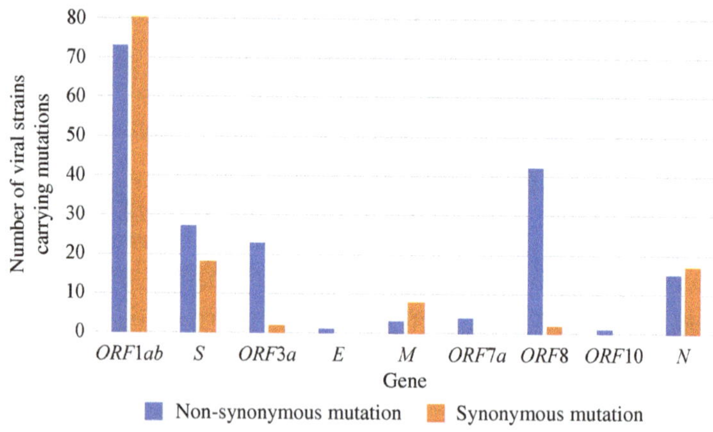

Figure 4-3.   Distribution of the numbers of strains carrying synonymous and non-synonymous mutations in different genes

2020, 97 SARS-CoV-2 genome sequences had been reported, among which 32 sequences (33.0%) did not have non-synonymous mutations, and the majority of the sequences (65 strains, 67%) only had one or two amino acid changes. There were 26 strains (26.8%) carrying the ORF8 L84S mutation. Tracing the genomic data, we found that the number of these mutant strains rapidly grew between January 14 and 31, and the strains carrying the ORF7a P34S mutation, the second most prevalent mutant strain, plateaued in their number, if not decreased. Based on extant data, the mutant strain with ORF8 L84S has significantly higher frequency than those with ORF7a P34S. The high prevalence of the strain indicates its probable high transmissibility if the cause by clustered transmissions can be excluded by further evidence. This suggests a need for close monitoring of the mutant strain.

4.3 Impact of Mutations on Clinical Pathogenic Diagnoses

To clinically diagnose SARS-CoV-2 infection through nucleic acid detection kits, primers and probes targeting the *ORF1ab* and *N* genes are recommended.

Based on WHO guidelines, when designing sets of primers and probes, N3 is used for general detection of SARS-like coronaviruses, and N1 and N2 are used for specific detection of SARS-CoV-2. The mutation sites reported in the *N* gene are $18C \to T$, $415T \to C$, $443C \to T$, $519A \to T$, $576C \to T$, $581C \to T$, $605G \to A$, $746A \to T$, $822C \to T$, $927C \to T$, $1030C \to T$, and $1176C \to T$. Among these mutations, the first three are located within N1 or N3, where the region is used for designing primers and probes used in real-time polymerase chain reaction (RT-PCR). Even though each of these three mutations was only detected in one strain of virus, we still advise caution against possible false negatives caused by them (Table 4-1).

The *ORF1ab* gene region has 99 reported mutated sites, none of which are covered by the target regions for the designed primers or probes (13076 – 13194 or 18512 – 18643; Table 4-2). In our

Table 4-1. Sequences and target regions of the RT-PCR primers based on *N* gene for detecting SARS-CoV-2. The letter F, R, and P stand for forward primers, reverse primers, and fluorescent probes, respectively.

Source of primers		Sequence	Target region	Reported mutations
WHO _N1	F	5′-GACCCCAAAATCAGCGAAAT-3′	13–84	18C→T
	R	5′-TCTGGTTACTGCCAGTTGAATCTG-3′		
	P	5′-FAM-ACCCCGCATTACGTTTGGTGGA CC-BHQ1-3′		
WHO _N2	F	5′-TTACAAACATTGGCCGCAAA-3′	890–956	None
	R	5′-GCGCGACATTCCGAAGAA-3′		
	P	5′-FAM-ACAATTTGCCCCCAGCGCTTC AG-BHQ1-3′		
WHO _N3	F	5′-GGGAGCCTTGAATACACCAAAA-3′	407–478	415T→C 443C→T
	R	5′-TGTAGCACGATTGCAGCATTG-3′		
	P	5′-FAM-AYCACATTGGCACCCGCAATCC TG-BQH1-3′		
China CDC	F	5′-GGGGAACTTCTCCTGCTAGAAT-3′	607–705	None
	R	5′-CAGACATTTTGCTCTCAAGCTG-3′		
	P	5′-FAM-TTGCTGCTGCTTGACAGATT- TARMA-3′		
Hong Kong	F	5′-TAATCAGACAAGGAACTGATTA-3′	871–980	None
	R	5′-CGAAGGTGTGACTTCCATG-3′		
	P	5′-FAM-GCAATTGTGCAATTTGCGG- TARMA-3′		

opinion, it is highly important and urgent to continue the sequencing studies of the viral genome, especially the constant monitoring of the aforementioned genetic mutations.

4.4 Impact of Mutations on Antigen Epitopes

By the end of February 2020, sequence analyses have revealed a total of 17 missense mutations on *S* gene; Figure 4-4 shows their detailed

Table 4-2. Sequences and target regions of the RT-PCR primers based on *ORF1ab* gene for detecting SARS-CoV-2. The letter F, R, and P stand for forward primers, reverse primers, and fluorescent probes, respectively.

Source of primers		Sequence	Target region	Reported mutations
China CDC	F	5′-CCCTGTGGGTTTTACACTTAA-3′	13076	None
	R	5′-ACGATTGTGCATCAGCTGA-3′	—	
	P	5′-FAM-CCGTCTGCGGTATGTGGAAAGGTTAT GG-BHQ1-3′	13194	
Hong Kong	F	5′-TGGGGYTTTACRGGTAACCT-3′	18512	None
	R	5′-AACRCGCTTAACAAAGCACTC-3′	—	
	P	5′-FAM-TAGTTGTGATGCWATCATGACTAG- BHQ1-3′	18643	

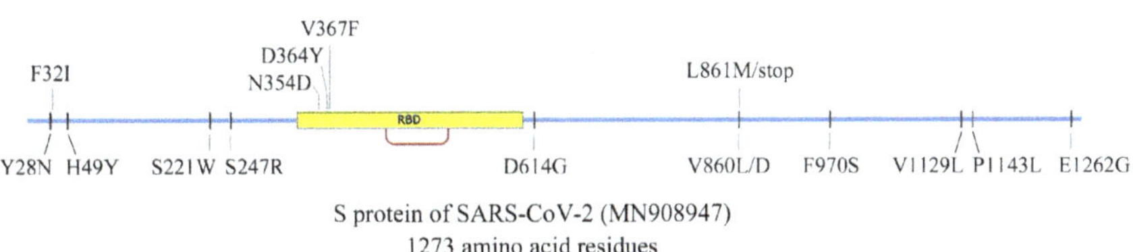

Figure 4-4. Distribution of missense mutations in S protein of SARS-CoV-2. Amino acid codes are based on the sequence of NCBI MN908947

mutation types. These mutations are all located outside of the antigen-recognition region, so we predict that they do not affect the binding of S protein and ACE2. Among them, one strain of virus exhibits a premature stop of translation (L861stop), which may substantially impact the function of S protein and calls for further studies.

Chapter 5
Mechanism of Infecting Host Cells

5.1 Targets and Mechanism of Viral Entry

Viral entry is the initial stage at which viruses infect a cell and one of the essential stages for transmission across species. This is no exception for viruses in the *Betacoronavirus* genus, including SARS-CoV-2. The genomes of SARS-CoV-2 and all other coronaviruses encode an important surface glycoprotein—S protein, which binds to the host cell receptor and mediates their entry into the cell. For viruses in the *Betacoronavirus* genus, the functional domain in which S protein mediates the binding to host cells is referred to as the receptor-binding domain (RBD). When RBD binds to the receptor, the protease of the host often initiates hydrolysis of the S protein, enabling the release of the spike fusion polypeptide and thereby further promoting viral entry. ACE2 is the host receptor of SARS-CoV-2, which is the same as that of SARS-CoV, while the host receptor of MERS-CoV is dipeptidyl peptidase 4 (DPP4, also known as CD26).

Previous studies on SARS-CoV show that the RBD of S protein is able to spontaneously complete structural folding and bind to the host receptor independent of other regions on the S protein. For instance, by replacing the RBD of the S protein in bat-derived Betacoronavirus Rp3, the resulting virions can enter transgenic mouse cells that express human ACE2, completing the cross-species transmission of the virus. This may be one of the reasons for the controversies over the origin of SARS-CoV-2. It also underscores the importance of the RBD in S protein. On January 22, 2020, by recombining the *RBD* gene of S protein into an engineered vector *in vitro*, scientists confirmed that the RBD of SAR-CoV-2 could bind to and enter the cells that express human *ACE2* gene, instead of DPP4 or human aminopeptidase N (APN), the known receptors of other Betacoronaviruses.

In animal models, SARS-CoV-2 can infect mice by entering cells through transgenic human-ACE2. Infecting human ACE2 (hACE2) transgenic mice and wild-type mice respectively with SARS-CoV-2 in 10^5 Median Tissue Culture Infective Dose ($TCID_{50}$) intranasally, focal lesions were observed in the right middle lung lobe of the infected hACE2 mice after 3 days. At the same time, the lung tissues of hACE2 mice exhibited mild or moderate multifocal pneumonia with interstitial hyperplasia, which was not observed in the wild-type mice infected with the virus or in the hACE2 mice of the uninfected control group (Figure 5–1). Consistently, the viral RNA was detected in the lung tissues of the SARS-CoV-2-infected hACE2 mice, but not in the other two groups. Furthermore, ten days after the inoculation, the infected hACE2 mice group lost 5% of their body weight, while the other two groups did not lose any weight. More convincingly, the immunofluorescent co-localization of the SARS-CoV-2 S protein and hACE2 was observed in alveolar epithelial cells of the infected hACE2 mice.

Therefore, SARS-CoV-2 has been confirmed to enter cells and infect the host by binding to hACE2 in both transgenic cell and transgenic mouse models.

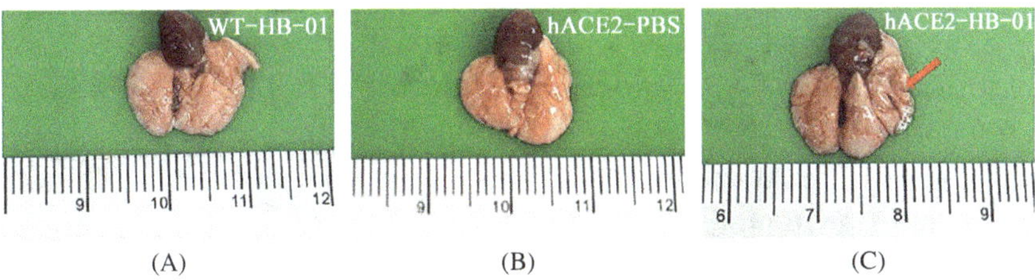

Figure 5-1. Gross pathology of the lungs in the mouse models **A**: SARS-CoV-2-infected wild-type mouse; **B**: Mock-infected hACE2 mouse inoculated with an equivalent volume of PBS, as a control; **C**: SARS-CoV-2-infected hACE2 mouse. (Bao LL, Deng W, Huang BY, *et al*. The pathogenicity of 2019 novel coronavirus in hACE2 transgenic mice. *bioRxiv*. (2020–02–07) [2020–02–23]. https://doi.org/10.1101/2020.02.07.939389.)

5.2 Structural Analysis of the S Protein

Scientists in the United States analyzed the prefusion conformation of the S protein trimers in SARS-CoV-2 with a resolution of 3.5 Å with cryo-electron microscopy. The results show that the structure of this protein is very similar to those of S proteins in SARS-CoV and MERS-CoV. In these three viruses, all the RBD structures exhibit a hinged conformation movement pattern to conceal or expose the key sites for receptor-binding. Unlike those of SARS-CoV and MERS-CoV, the RBD of SARS-CoV-2 is closer to the central part of the trimer. In an upward helical way, one of the RBDs in the trimer changes the spatial conformation of the S protein to bind to the host ACE2 (green part in the middle of Figure 5-2) more easily. Therefore, it has a higher affinity to the host ACE2 than the other two viruses. The biophysical and structural computation results show that the affinity of the SARS-CoV-2 S protein for human ACE2 is much higher than that of the SARS-CoV (>10–20 times), which explains the high infectivity of COVID-19 this time.

The S protein of Bat-CoV-RaTG13 is the closest to that of SARS-CoV-2 in homology, which is as high as 96% in their amino acid sequence. In the S protein of SARS-CoV-2, the protease cleavage site at the juncture of S1/S2 subunits is –RRAR– (furin protease recognition site, –RXXR–), different from those of SARS-CoV and Bat-CoV-RaTG13, which only have a single arginine residue. This insertion of the furin recognition site will increase the protease cleavage efficiency. Compared with the sequence of SARS-CoV, it is speculated from the structure that the inserted –SPRR– located at the amino acid residue position 680–683 is the most suitable substrate for transmembrane serine proteases (TMPRSSs). It can increase the enzyme cleavage efficiency of the two subunits in S protein, thus further promoting and enhancing the infectivity of SARS-CoV-2. Results from a single-cell transcriptome study also confirm the high co-expression of TMPRSSs and ACE2 in absorptive intestinal epithelial cells, esophageal epithelial cells, and alveolar type II (ATII) cells, suggesting the important role of TMPRSSs in viral infection. Similar furin protease recognition sites are also common in other influenza viruses with high virulence and is usually associated with the viral infection efficiency.

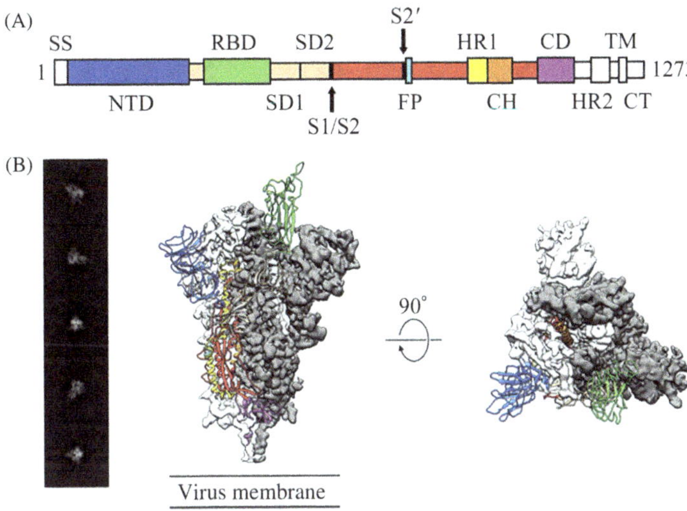

Figure 5-2. Binding structure of the SARS-CoV-2 S protein **A**: The primary structure schematic of the SARS-CoV-2 S protein, color coding according to the various domains. White is the region excluded from ectodomain expression constructs or invisible in the final schematic, and the arrows indicate protease cleavage sites. SS, signal sequence; NTD, N-terminal domain; RBD, receptor-binding domain; SD1, sub-structural domain 1; SD2, sub-structural domain 2; S1/S2, S1/S2 protease cleavage sites; S2′, S2′ protease cleavage sites; FP, fusion peptide; HR1, heptapeptide repeated sequence 1; CH, central helix; CD, connected domain; HR2, heptapeptide repeated sequence 2; TM, transmembrane domain; CT, cytoplasmic tail. **B**: Select 2D class averages of the particles used for calculating the reconstruction of the SARS-CoV-2 S protein (*left*). Side and top views of the prefusion structure of the SARS-CoV-2 S protein, with a single RBD in an "up" conformation (*right*). The two RBD "down" promotors display as cryo-EM density in either white or grey, and the color of the RBD "up" promotor corresponds to the schematic in panel A. (Yan RH, Zhang YY, Guo YY, *et al*. Structural basis for the recognition of the 2019-nCoV by human ACE2. *bioRxiv*. (2020–02–19) [2020–02–23]. https://doi.org/10.1101/2020.02.19.956946.)

In addition to the amino acid differences at the juncture of the S1/S2 subunits, there are 29 amino acid differences between the S proteins of SARS-CoV-2 and that of Bat-CoV-RaTG13, among which 17 are located in the RBD.

A research team from Westlake University also analyzed the structure of the SARS-CoV-2 RBD bound to the full length human ACE2 protein with cryo-electron microscopy. Their structure shows that the extracellular peptidase domain (PD) in each ACE2 protein can bind to the RBD

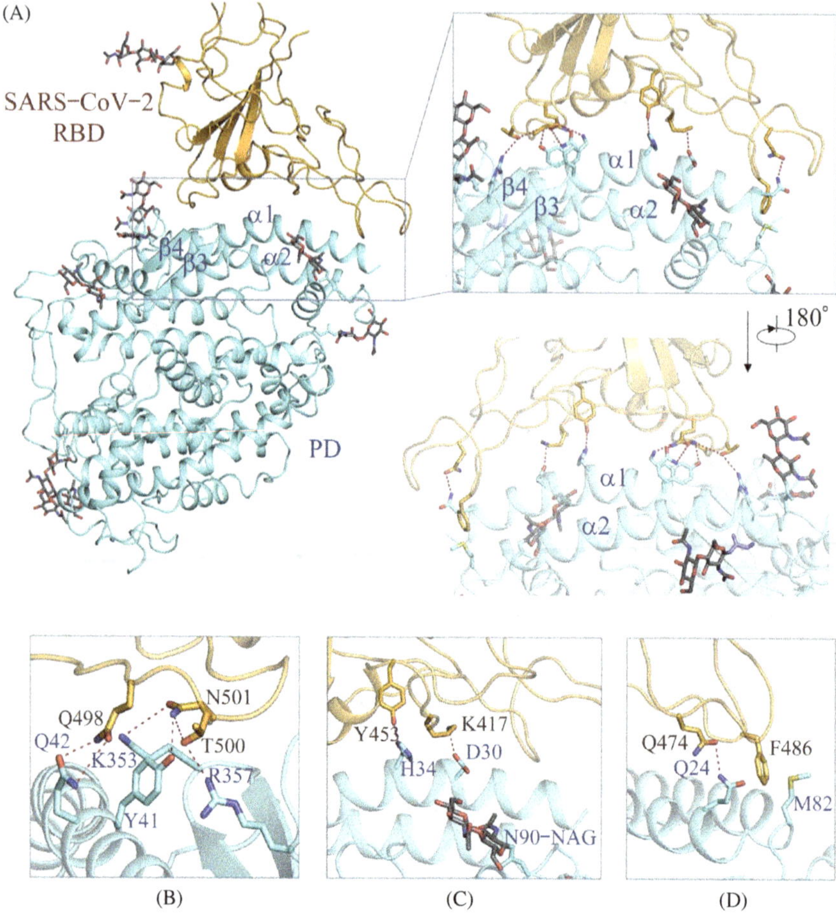

Figure 5-3. The interactions between SARS-CoV-2 RBD and ACE2 **A**: PD in ACE2 mainly binds with the α1 helix when it identifies RBD. The α2 helix and the linker between β3 and β4 also contribute to the interaction. This figure shows only one RBD–ACE2. **B–D**: The detailed analysis of the interface between SARS-CoV-2 RBD and ACE2. Polar interactions are indicated by red dashed lines. (Yan RH, Zhang YY, Guo YY, *et al*. Structural basis for the recognition of the 2019-nCoV by human ACE2. *bioRxiv*. (2020–02–19) [2020–02–23]. https://doi.org/10.1101/2020.02.19.956946.)

of an S protein, and their binding is mainly through polar interaction, which is similar to the binding of the SARS-CoV RBD to ACE2.

A loop extending outward in RBD spans over the arched α1 helix of ACE2 protein like a bridge (Figure 5-3A), meanwhile, the α2 helix and the loop connecting β3 and β4 barrels also play important roles in stabilizing the binding of RBD and ACE2. Specifically, the interactions between RBD and PD can be divided into three clusters. At the left of the "bridge" is the N-terminal of the α1 helix, where a hydrogen bond (H-bond) network is formed between the Gln498, Thr500, and Asn501 in RBD, and the Tyr41, Gln42, Lys353, and Arg357 in ACE2 (Figure 5-3B). In the middle of the "bridge", the Lys417 and Tyr453 in RBD respectively interact with the Asp30 and His34 in ACE2 (Figure 5-3C). On the right of the "bridge" is the C-terminal of the α1 helix, where H-bonds are formed between Gln474 in RBD and Gln24 in ACE2, while Phe486 in RBD interacts with Met82 in ACE2 through van der Waals force (Figure 5-3D). In these RBDs, most of the residues critical to the binding of ACE2 are highly conserved or have similar characteristics to those in the SARS-CoV RBD. The similarity in structure and sequence suggests that convergent evolution may occur in RBDs of SARS-CoV-2 and of SARS-CoV, thereby further strengthening their binding to ACE2.

The structural analyses of ACE2 and SARS-CoV-2 RBD have deepened our understanding of the mechanism of virus infection, guiding future efforts in target drug and diagnostic tools development.

5.3 Expression of the ACE2 Gene and Infection Sites

After confirming the host receptor for SARS-CoV-2, another important medical and scientific question pertains to the organs targeted by the virus. In addition to the respiratory system, clinical data indicated that the great majority of COVID-19 patients exhibited varying degrees of liver and kidney damage, which may be associated with the high expression of the *ACE2* gene in these organs. Multiple research teams studied the expression levels of *ACE2* gene in human organs and tissues. They found that organs such as the lung, heart, esophagus, kidney, bladder, and ileum are at high risk of SARS-CoV-2 infection. In these organs, cells such as alveolar type II cells, cardiomyocytes, renal proximal tubular cells, ileal and esophageal epithelial cells, and urothelial cells of the bladder are especially susceptible to viral infection. A team by Professor Lan Fei from Fudan University-Affiliated

Zhongshan Hospital has confirmed the specific high expression of *ACE2* gene in bile duct cells of healthy population through single-cell RNA-seq, suggesting that the liver damage by viral infection may have resulted from the dysfunction of bile duct cells or immunological liver damage, rather than the damage of hepatocytes directly caused by the virus. Furthermore, researchers in both China and the US have reported the highest expression of *ACE2* gene in male testis, including the Leydig cells, seminiferous tubular cells, and renal tubular cells, suggesting that SARS-CoV-2 is very likely to give rise to testicular damage and subsequent male infertility. This is consistent with the symptoms of orchitis reported in some male patients clinically.

5.4 Life Cycle of the Coronaviruses

The complete cycle for the coronavirus infecting a cell includes: viral entry, replication–transcription, and viral shedding. Since the replication and shedding of SARS-CoV-2 are rarely reported, here we take SARS-CoV as an example to introduce the replication of coronaviruses under the same genus (Figure 5-4).

5.4.1 *Viral entry*

The S protein on the surface of SARS-CoV specifically binds to the host ACE2, triggering the fusion of the viral outer membrane with the cellular membrane or endosomal membrane. Upon entering the cell through endocytosis, the virus releases its genomic positive-sense RNA ((+)RNA) into the cytoplasm. Since the mechanism of viral entry for SARS-CoV-2 has been described in detail earlier in this chapter, we will not repeat it here.

5.4.2 *Replication–transcription*

The process of viral replication–transcription is as follows.

(1) The genomic (+)RNA is translated into polyprotein1a (pp1a) and polyprotein1ab (pp1ab). Then, the NSP3 and NSP5 protease domains in pp1a recognize the specific amino acid sites in these

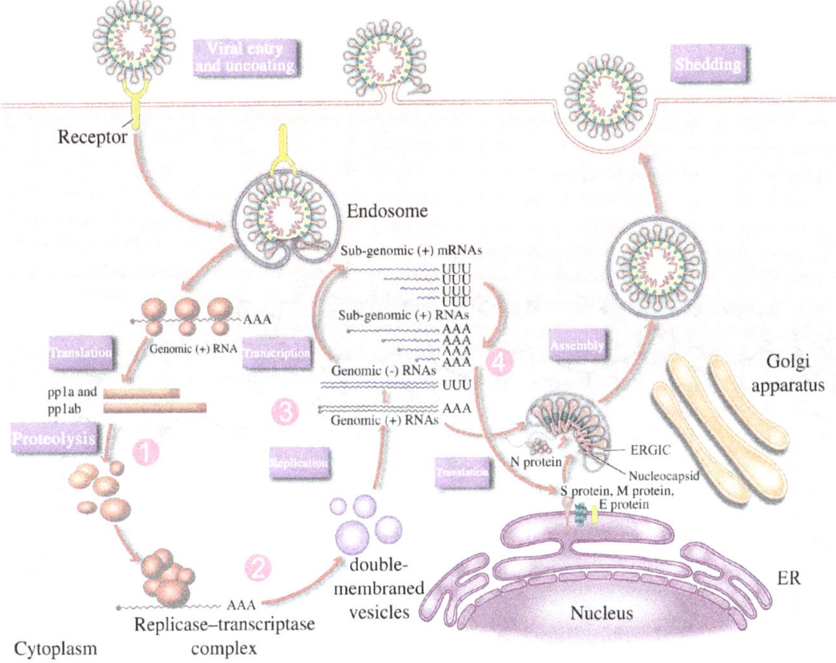

Figure 5-4. Schematic of SARS-CoV replication

Note: (1) The assembly of replicase–transcriptase complex by NSP1 – 16. (2) The assembly of replication–transcription complex. (3) Virus replication. (4) Transcription and translation of structural and accessory proteins. ER: endoplasmic reticulum; ERGIC: endoplasmic reticulum-Golgi intermediate compartment. This schematic is adapted from de Wit E, van Doremalen N, Falzarano D, *et al.* SARS and MERS: recent insights into emerging coronaviruses. *Nat Rev Microbiol.* 2016;14(8):523-534.

polyproteins and eventually cleave them into NSP1 — 16. These NSPs are subsequently assembled into the replicase–transcriptase complex.

(2) Replication–transcription complexes (RTC) are assembled from the replicase–transcriptase–genomic (+)RNA complexes and membrane structures derived from the rough endoplasmic reticulum (RER).

(3) Inside the RTCs, NSP12 — the RNA replicase — produces double-stranded RNA with the (+)RNA as the template, during which the exonuclease NSP14 proofreads the replication.

(4) The double-stranded RNA is transcribed into 12 sub-genomic RNAs of varying lengths, which are then translated into S, M, E, N, and accessory proteins.

5.4.3 *Viral shedding*

The newly synthesized (+)RNAs are enveloped by N proteins and RER structures embedded with S, M, and E proteins, assembling into viral particles. These viral particles are then excreted through the Golgi apparatus pathway and become mature progeny virions.

References

1. Geng HY, Tan WJ. Research progress of the newly discovered coronavirus. [Chinese]. *Chin J Virol.* 2013;(1):65–70.
2. Alagaili AN, Briese T, Mishra N, *et al.* Middle East respiratory syndrome coronavirus infection in dromedary camels in Saudi Arabia. *mBio.* 2014;5(2):e01002–14.
3. Alexander EG, Susan CB, Ralph SB, *et al.* Severe acute respiratory syndrome-related coronavirus: The species and its viruses-a statement of the Coronavirus Study Group. *bioRxiv.* (2020–02–11) [2020–02–23]. https://doi.org/10.1101/2020.02.07.937862.
4. Bao LL, Deng W, Huang BY, *et al.* The pathogenicity of 2019 novel coronavirus in hACE2 transgenic mice. *bioRxiv.* (2020–02–07) [2020–02–23]. https://doi.org/10.1101/2020.02.07.939389.
5. Becker MW, Graham RL, Donaldson EF, *et al.* Synthetic recombinant bat SARS-like coronavirus is infectious in cultured cells and in mice. *Proc Natl Acad Sci USA.* 2008;105(50),19944–19949.
6. Chan JF, Yuan S, Kok KH, *et al.* A familial cluster of pneumonia associated with the 2019 novel coronavirus indicating person-to-person transmission: a study of a family cluster. *Lancet.* 2020;395(10223):514–523.
7. Chan JF, Kok KH, Zhu Z, *et al.* Genomic characterization of the 2019 novel human-pathogenic coronavirus isolated from a patient with atypical pneumonia after visiting Wuhan. *Emerg Microbes Infect.* 2020;9(1): 221–236.
8. de Wit E, van Doremalen N, Falzarano D, *et al.* SARS and MERS: recent insights into emerging coronaviruses. *Nat Rev Microbiol.* 2016;14(8): 523–534.

9. Fehr AR, Perlman S. Coronaviruses: An overview of their replication and pathogenesis. *Methods Mol Biol.* 2015;1282:1–23.

10. Lam TY, Shum MH, Zhu HC, *et al.* Identification of 2019-nCoV related coronaviruses in Malayan pangolins in southern China. *bioRxiv.* (2020–02–13) [2020–02–23]. http://doi.org/10.1101/2020.02.13.945485.

11. Li F, Li W, Farzan M, *et al.* Structure of SARS coronavirus spike receptor binding domain complexed with receptor [J]. *Science.* 2005;309(5742): 1864–1868.

12. Liu P, Chen W, Chen JP. Viral metagenomics revealed sendai virus and coronavirus infection of Malayan pangolins (*Manis javanica*) [J]. *Viruses.* 2019;11(11):979.

13. Lu R, Zhao X, Li J, *et al.* Genomic characterization and epidemiology of 2019 novel coronavirus: implications for virus origins and receptor binding. *Lancet.* 2020;395(10224):565–574.

14. Letko M, Munster V. Functional assessment of cell entry and receptor usage for lineage B β-coronaviruses, including 2019-nCoV. *bioRxiv.* (2020–01–22) [2020–02–23]. http://doi.org/10.1101/2020.01.22.915660.

15. Ogando NS, Ferron F, Decroly E, *et al.* The curious case of the nidovirus exoribonuclease: Its role in RNA synthesis and replication fidelity. *Front Microbiol.* 2019;10(1813):1–17.

16. Su S, Wong G, Shi W, *et al.* Epidemiology, genetic recombination, and pathogenesis of coronaviruses. *Trends Microbiol.* 2016;24(6):490–502.

17. Wahba L, Jain N, Fire AZ, *et al.* Identification of a pangolin niche for a 2019-nCoV-like coronavirus through an extensive meta-metagenomic search. *bioRxiv.* (2020–02–08) [2020–02–23]. http://doi.org/10.1101/2020.02.08.939660.

18. Wong MC, Javornik Cregeen SJ, Ajami NJ, *et al.* Evidence of recombination in coronaviruses implicating pangolin origins of nCoV-2019. *bioRxiv.* (2020–02–07) [2020–02–23]. http://doi.org/10.1101/2020.02.07.939207.

19. Wrapp D, Wang N, Corbett KS, *et al.* Cryo-EM structure of the 2019-nCoV spike in the prefusion conformation. *Science.* 2020;367(6483):1260–1263.

20. Wu AP, Peng YS, Huang BY, *et al.* Genome composition and divergence of the novel coronavirus (2019-nCoV) originating in China. *Cell Host Microbe.* 2020;27(3):325–328.

21. Wu F, Zhao S, Yu B, *et al.* A new coronavirus associated with human respiratory disease in China. *Nature.* 2020;579:265–269.

22. Xiao K, Zhai J, Feng Y, *et al.* Isolation and characterization of 2019-nCoV-like coronavirus from Malayan pangolins. *bioRxiv.* (2020–02–17) [2020–02–23]. http://doi.org/10.1101/2020.02.17.951335.

23. Zhang LL, Lin DZ, Sun XY, *et al*. X-ray structure of main protease of the novel coronavirus SRAS-CoV-2 enables design of α-Ketoamide inhibitors. *bioRxiv*. (2020–02–17) [2020–02–23]. https://doi.org/10.1101/2020.02.17.952879.

24. Zhou P, Yang XL, Wang XG, *et al*. A pneumonia outbreak associated with a new coronavirus of probable bat origin. *Nature*. 2020;579:270–273.

25. Zhu N, Zhang D, Wang W, *et al*. A novel coronavirus from patients with pneumonia in China, 2019. *N Engl J Med*. 2020;382(8):727–733.

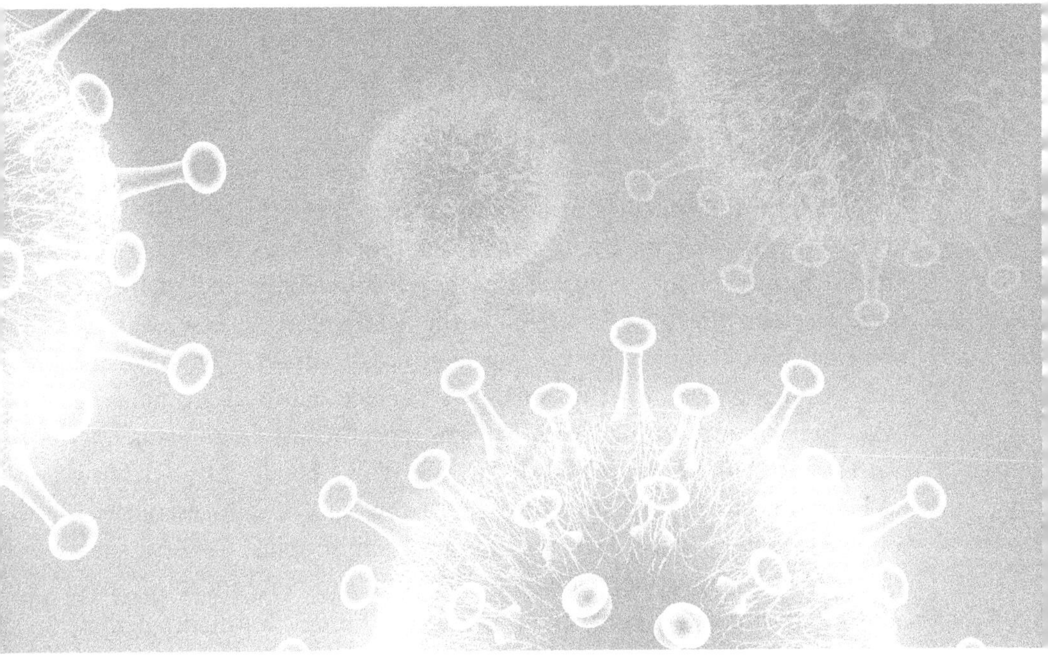

Part 3

Immunology and Vaccine Development

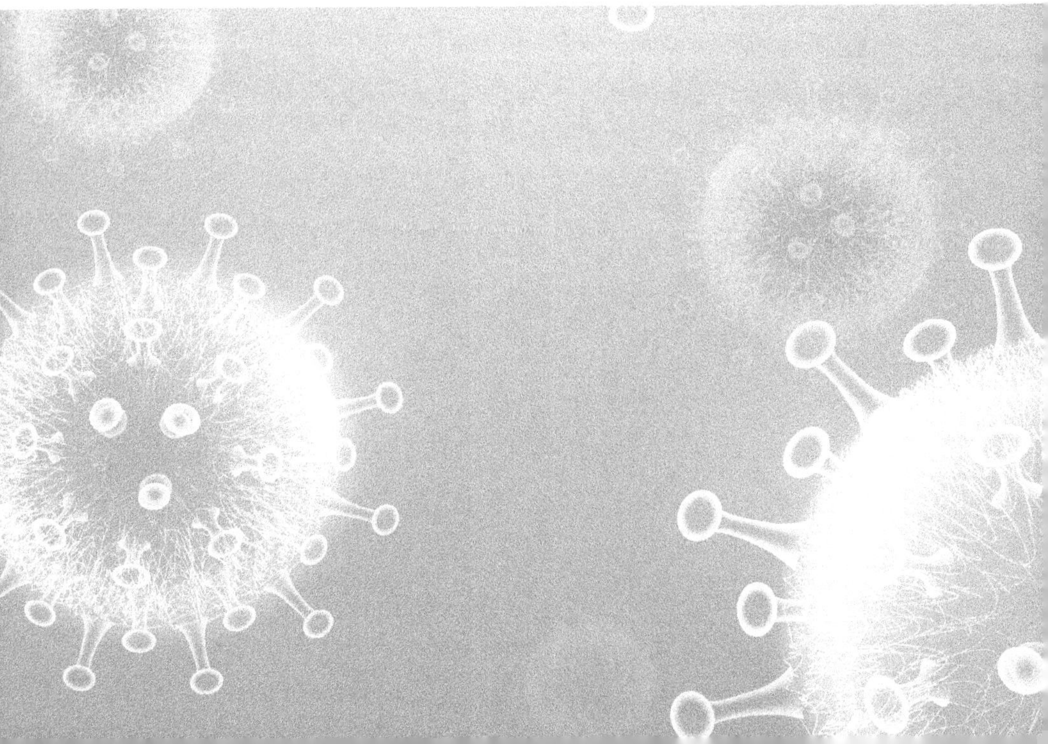

The invention of vaccines marks a milestone in the history of human development. Looking back, many infectious diseases that have devastated humanity for centuries are now almost eradicated thanks to their vaccines. Smallpox, a highly virulent infectious disease, was the first one to be completely eradicated in human history. The invention and popularization of the smallpox vaccine allowed humans to develop immunity to the smallpox virus, and the last case of smallpox was recorded in 1978. In May 1980, the World Health Organization (WHO) declared that smallpox had been successfully eradicated. Similarly, many other infectious diseases such as polio, mumps, measles, rubella, tetanus, pertussis, diphtheria, hepatitis A, and rinderpest have been effectively controlled following the development of their vaccines, and some are even almost eradicated.

The existing evidence confirms that SARS-CoV-2 has intermediate hosts. For the viruses with natural intermediate hosts, even if the epidemic can be effectively controlled by isolation and treatment, having a vaccine is still the most cost-efficient, effective, and lasting prevention and control measure against the recurrence of large-scale outbreaks. This section is dedicated to the current research on the immunology and vaccinology of SARS-CoV-2, as well as the vaccines of other coronaviruses.

Chapter 6
Progress in Immunology Research

6.1 Research Targeting the S Protein

SARS-CoV-2 is a positive-sense single-stranded RNA coronavirus. Its genome encodes four major viral structural proteins (Figure 6-1): S, E, M, and N proteins. Among them, the M and E proteins play important roles in viral assembly, while the N protein is necessary for RNA synthesis. The S protein is responsible for binding with the receptor to mediate the viral entry to host cells, and its receptor-binding domain (RBD) is a key target for neutralizing antibodies, rendering the S protein a major therapeutic target.

The S protein in coronaviruses mediates the viral entry to host cells by binding to the cell receptor; its RBD is a key target for neutralizing antibodies. Therefore, it is widely-recognized that the S protein is one of the most promising targets for the development of coronavirus vaccines (Figure 6-1). The RBDs in SARS-CoV-2 and in SARS-CoV have high homology. A research group led by Dr. Ying Tianlei at Fudan University discovered that the S protein of SARS-CoV-2 had cross-reactivity with the antibody against SARS-CoV, which is of great significance to the development of SARS-CoV-2 vaccines and its therapeutic antibodies. Enzyme-linked immunosorbent assay (ELISA) and biolayer interferometry binding (BLI) were applied to verify that CR3022, a specific human monoclonal antibody of SARS-CoV, can bind effectively to the RBD of SARS-CoV-2, as well as recognize an epitope different from the binding site of ACE2.

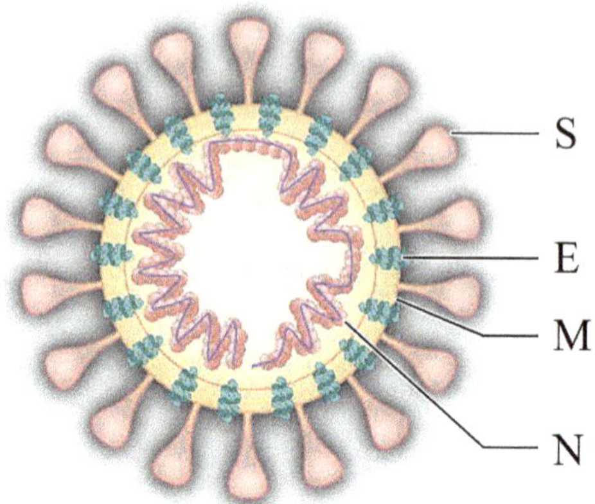

Figure 6-1. Schematic of the structure of SARS-CoV-2

Note: S, spike; E, envelope; M, membrane; N, nucleocapsid

Their results indicate that CR3022 may be administered either independently or synergistically with other neutralizing antibodies for the prevention and treatment of SARS-CoV-2 infection.

The S2 subunit of the S protein in SARS-CoV plays a critical role in regulating viral fusion. The HR1 and HR2 domains can form a six-helical bundle (6-HB) to enable the fusion of the virus to the cellular membrane. International researchers designed SARS-CoV-2-HR1P and SARS-CoV-2-HR2P, two fusion inhibitors targeting S-HR1 and S-HR2, respectively. They found that SARS-CoV-2-HR2P could inhibit the fusion between SARS-CoV-2 and the target host cell. At the same time, they also confirmed that both the pan-coronavirus fusion inhibitors EK1 and SARS-CoV-2-HR2P showed strong inhibitory activities on both the cellular fusion mediated by S protein and the pseudovirus infection of SARS-CoV-2. These results suggest that the HR1 and HR2 regions in SARS-CoV-2 can be candidate targets for the development of SARS-CoV-2 fusion inhibitors.

Cross-reactive epitopes (CREs) are consensus or similar epitope regions on the surface of antigens across multiple viruses. These regions can be bound or neutralized by the same antibodies. Some scholars use CE-BLAST to compute antigenic similarities to study the

S antigens in other coronaviruses that are similar to that in SARS-CoV-2. The higher the similarity, the more likely cross-reactions would occur between the paired antigens. This study found that SARS-CoV-2 and SARS-CoV had a high similarity in the ACE2-binding sites on S proteins (the similarity score was higher than 0.8, with a default cutoff of 0.75), suggesting the existence of potential CREs shared by the two coronaviruses. This result inspires new approaches for the development of SARS-CoV-2 vaccines.

6.2 Antigen Epitope Prediction

The E protein is a transmembrane protein. It plays multiple major or auxiliary roles in the life cycles of several coronaviruses, such as envelope formation, assembly, and budding. Moreover, it interacts with other viral structural proteins (M, N, and S proteins) and proteins in the host cell (Figure 6-2).

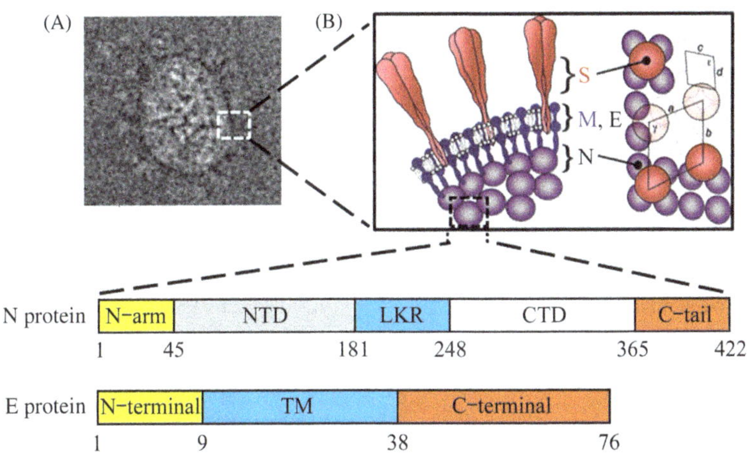

Figure 6-2.   Schematic of the structures of N Proteins and E proteins in SARS-CoV. **A**: Two-dimensional reconstructed electron microscope image of SARS-CoV. **B**: Domains of N protein and E protein

Note: NTD, N-terminal domain; LKR, linker region; CTD, C-terminal domain; TM, transmembrane domain; S, spike protein; M, membrane protein; E, envelope protein. (Chang CK, Hou MH, Chang CF, *et al.* The SARS coronavirus nucleocapsid protein-forms and functions. *Antiviral Res.* 2014;103:39-50.)

Some international research institutes predicted the potential targets for synthetic peptide vaccines based on the structure of E protein. The core mechanism of synthetic peptide vaccines is the chemical synthesis of B-cell or T-cell epitopes that are immunodominant and can induce specific immune responses, both of which need to be coupled with a vector scaffold molecule. Such vaccines have advantages over others in that they do not require *in vitro* culturing, have high safety, and can activate accurate immune responses. Selecting the E protein as the immunogenic target, the study leveraged immunoinformatics and comparative genomic methods, as well as consulted the world population coverage. They identified ten MHC I-related peptides and ten MHC II-related peptides as potential targets of T cell epitope-based peptide vaccines designed for SARS-CoV-2 (Table 6-1). However, synthetic peptide vaccines usually lack sufficient immunogenicity, rendering it difficult to induce multiple immune responses as protein antigens do. Additionally, despite their theoretical properties, follow-up experiments are needed to determine their immunogenicity and safety.

N protein is the only protein that binds to the RNA genome of the coronavirus. It is involved in viral replication and the host

Table 6-1. Predicted T cell epitope-based peptides for SARS-CoV-2, with E protein as the target

MHC class-I epitopes-based peptide	MHC class-II epitopes-based peptide
57–YVYSRVKNL–65	53–KPSFYVYSRVKNLNS–67
50–SLVKPSFYV–58	52–VKPSFYVYSRVKNLN–66
16–SVLLFLAFV–24	51–LVKPSFYVYSRVKNL–65
20–FLAFVVFLL–28	54–PSFYVYSRVKNLNSS–68
17–VLLFLAFVV–25	45–NIVNVSLVKPSFYVY–59
38–RLCAYCCNI–46	27–LLVTLAILTALRLCA–41
4–FVSEETGTL–12	55–SFYVYSRVKNLNSSR–69
34–LTALRLCAY–42	28–LVTLAILTALRLCAY–42
51–LVKPSFYVY–59	29–VTLAILTALRLCAYC–43
45–NIVNVSLVK–53	44–CNIVNVSLVKPSFYV–58

Table 6-2. The predicted T cell epitopes for SARS-CoV-2, with N protein and surface glycoprotein as targets

Target	MHC class-I epitope	MHC class-II epitope
N protein	119–AGLPYGANK–127	289–QELIRQGTDYKH–300
		291–LIRQGTDYKHWP–302
	397–AADLDDFSK–405	226–RLNQLESKMSGK–237
		227–LNQLESKMSGKG–238
	229–QLESKMSGK–237	224–LDRLNQLESKMS–235
Surface glycoprotein	975–SVLNDILSR–983	315–TSNFRVQPTESI–326
	550–GVLTESNKK–558	316–SNFRVQPTESIV–327
	454–RLFRKSNLK–462	117–LLIVNNATNVVI–128
	409–QIAPGQTGK–417	

response to viral infection. Using reverse vaccinology and immunoinformatics, based on the scores of antigens, an international research team screened out the epitopes that meet the requirements among those generated by the Immune Epitope Database (IEDB) server. They identified three MHC I epitopes and five MHC II epitopes targeting the N protein, as well as four MHC I epitopes and three MHC II epitopes targeting the surface glycoproteins (Table 6-2). Meanwhile, they performed peptide-protein docking to select top candidates and validated that all the epitopes can bind with MHC I or MHC II molecules. This suggests that all these molecules can bind to their corresponding targets and have the potential to induce immune responses. Furthermore, they selected non-allergenic and non-toxic epitopes with high antigenicity as core parts, paired with three different adjuvants (β-defensin, L7/L12 ribosomal protein, and HABA protein), and constructed three subunit vaccines (CV-1, CV-2, and CV-3) for SARS-CoV-2. By analyzing the antigenicity, allergenicity and physicochemical properties of these three vaccines, they found CV-1 to be the best candidate. Subsequent molecular dynamic simulations and *in silico* codon adaptation analyses were performed on CV-1. Their results showed that the TLR-8-CV-1 docked complex was very stable, with a codon adaptation index (CAI) of 1.0, indicating that the DNA sequence should have very high amount of

Table 6-3. The predicted CD4[+] T-cell epitopes for SARS-CoV-2, with S protein, E protein, and M protein as targets

Target	The predicted epitope
S protein	232–GINITRFQTLLALHR–246
	233–INITRFQTLLALHRS–247
E protein	55–SFYVYSRVKNLNSSR–69
	56–FYVYSRVKNLNSSRV–70
	57–YVYSRVKNLNSSRVP–71
M protein	97–IASFRLFARTRSMWS–111
	98–ASFRLFARTRSMWSF–112
	99–SFRLFARTRSMWSFN–113

favorable codons that should be able to express the desired amino acid in *Escherichia coli* strain K12. Therefore, the researchers believe that CV-1 can be produced in large quantities by fermenting in *E. coli* K12 on the vector pET-19b.

Through comprehensive experiments and computations, this study showed that these vaccines probably had good immunogenicity. If subsequent *in vitro* and *in vivo* experiments also yield promising results, these vaccine candidates are very likely to be used to prevent the transmission of SARS-CoV-2.

Separately, another research team has identified eight CD4[+] T-cell epitopes with high binding affinity (HBA), which are distributed in S protein ($n = 2$), E protein ($n = 3$) and M protein ($n = 3$), respectively. These epitopes can be generally identified by the *HLA-DR* alleles of the Asia-Pacific Region population and can be used as potential universal epitopes for the development of SARS-CoV-2 subunit vaccines (Table 6-3).

6.3 ACE2 Fusion Protein

Human ACE2 protein is the key functional receptor of SARS-CoV-2 infection. A research team in China has successfully constructed the recombinant ACE2 fusion protein (ACE2-Ig) by connecting the extracellular domain of human ACE2 and the Fc region of human

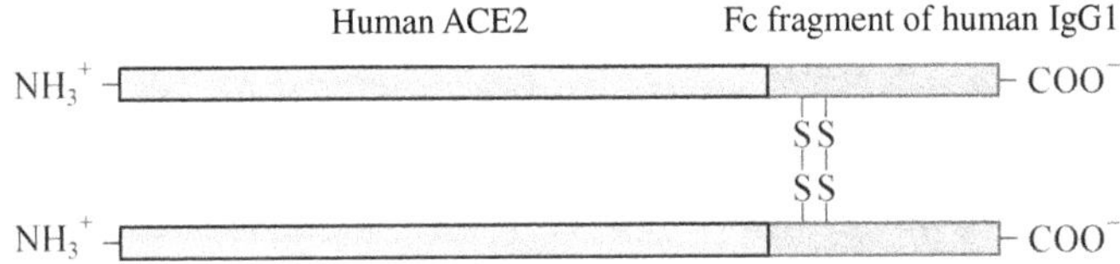

Figure 6-3. Schematic of ACE2-Ig

IgG1 (Figure 6-3). They showed that this fusion protein had a high affinity for RBDs of SARS-CoV and SARS-CoV-2 and could effectively neutralize SARS-CoV and SARS-CoV-2 *in vitro*. This fusion protein may be used as a research reagent to develop vaccines and virus inhibitors. However, ACE2 proteins have a relatively fast clearance rate in humans and mice. According to the pharmacokinetic reports, its half-life was only a few hours, which may become a hindrance to the application of human ACE2 protein.

6.4 T-Cell Exhaustion and Cytokine Storm

T cell exhaustion is a common feature in many chronic infections and tumors in both mice and humans. Due to long-term exposure to persistent antigens and inflammation, the initial T cells differentiate into exhausted T cells (TEX). TEX can restrict some immune responses against pathogen infections or tumors, thereby limiting immune-mediated pathological damages. However, this restrictive function often brings about the continuous progress and deterioration of the disease. A study reviewed 522 laboratory-confirmed COVID-19 patients admitted to hospitals from December 2019 to January 2020, examining their total counts of T cells, CD4⁺ T cells, and CD8⁺ T cells, as well as the patients' concentrations of serum cytokine. After testing the expression of TEX markers (programmed death-1 (PD-1)) and T cell immunoglobulin and mucin domain-3 (TIM-3) in the peripheral blood of 14 patients, the researchers discovered that the number of T cells in the peripheral blood of COVID-19 patients had declined significantly, with the remaining T cells exhibiting functional exhaustion.

Cytokine storm is a phenomenon of excessive inflammatory response caused by the rapid and massive production of cytokines upon microorganism infections. It is believed to be one of the causes for acute respiratory distress syndrome (ARDS) and multiple organ dysfunctions. In the reported cases of SARS, MERS, and COVID-19, cytokine storm was an important factor for deterioration of diseases and even death. The study showed that the counts of total T cells, CD4$^+$ T cells, and CD8$^+$ T cells were negatively correlated with the levels of tumor necrosis factor-á (TNF- á), IL-6, and IL-10. The source and the triggers of these cytokines are issues of concern. In the study, the researchers believed that these cytokines were not produced by T cells; on the contrary, a cytokine storm might accelerate the necrosis and apoptosis of T cells, resulting in a decreased number of T cells. Further studies are still required to understand whether SARS-CoV-2 also promotes the release of cytokines from monocytes and macrophages in COVID-19 patients.

Chapter 7
Research on Coronavirus Vaccines

7.1 The Research Strategy for Coronavirus Vaccines

As there has not been sufficient research on SARS-CoV-2 vaccines so far, we can draw inspiration from past research on vaccines against SARS-CoV and MERS-CoV (Table 7-1).

7.1.1 *Recombinant vector vaccine*

Currently, the viral vectors used to construct SARS-CoV or MERS-CoV recombinant vector vaccines are mainly adenovirus, poxvirus, and human parainfluenza virus (HPIV) vectors.

Adenoviruses are extensively used in light of its small genome structure (20 kb) and ease of manipulation. As live vectors, adenoviruses have a wide range of target cells, being able to infect not only dividing cells but also non-dividing cells. A research team has constructed two recombinant adenoviral vectors, encoding the full-length MERS-CoV S protein and its S1 extracellular domain, respectively. BALB/c mice were vaccinated through intramuscular injections and with subsequent secondary immunization boosted through intranasal inoculations three weeks afterward. It was shown that these two vaccines could both elicit MERS-CoV-specific immune responses in mice and allowed them to produce S-specific antibodies. The induced antibodies could neutralize MERS-CoV *in vitro*. Similarly, immunizing monkeys with adenovirus-based SARS vaccines

Table 7-1. Various types and characteristics of vaccines against SARS-CoV and MERS-CoV

Type of vaccine	Target	Vector/Adjuvant	Animal model
Recombinant vector vaccine	S protein	Human parainfluenza virus (HPIV)	African green monkey (*Cercopithecus aethiops*)
	S protein	Poxvirus (*Poxviridae*)	Laboratory mouse (*Mus musculus*) and Dromedary (*Camelus dromedarius*)
	S protein S1 subunit	Adenovirus (*Adenoviridae*)	Rhesus macaque (*Macaca mulatta*)
	M protein		
	N Protein		
RBD subunit vaccine	S protein RBD fragment	None	Laboratory mouse (*M. musculus*) and NZW rabbit (*Oryctolagus cuniculus*)
Adjuvant vaccine	S protein	Alum or MF59	Laboratory mouse (*M. musculus*)
	S protein RBD fragment	TLR4 (toll-like receptor 4) agonist	Laboratory mouse (*M. musculus*)

expressing S protein S1 subunit, M, and NP proteins could elicit strong protective neutralizing antibodies and T cell-mediated immune responses.

Poxviruses are widely used due to its desirable genomic stability, high expression levels, adequacy of non-essential genes, and capability of accommodating multiple foreign genes. Recombinant modified vaccinia virus Ankara (MVA) inoculated through intramuscular or subcutaneous injections could elicit high-level of MERS-CoV-specific neutralizing antibodies in BALB/c mice. Similarly, an MVA vaccine expressing the MERS-CoV spike protein could induce mucosal immunity in dromedaries (*Camelus dromedarius*). Three weeks after the boost immunization and subsequent intranasal inoculation of MERS-CoV, the dromedaries only exhibited mild clinical signs. In comparison with the control animals, these camels showed smaller rises in body temperature, had significantly lower mean viral titers, and significantly lower levels of infectious virus in excretion.

Some other researchers successfully constructed an attenuated HPIV coding the full-length S protein of SARS-CoV strain Urbani. The efficacy of the vaccine expressing SARS-CoV S protein was confirmed through vaccination of African green monkeys. However, the SARS-CoV vaccine based on full-length S protein could ultimately lead to severe adverse reactions like liver damage. It could also induce antibody-mediated disease enhancement (ADE) through the non-neutralizing epitopes of the S protein in the vaccinated animals. The safety and efficacy of such vaccines remain to be further investigated.

7.1.2 *RBD subunit vaccine*

Compared to other parts of the S protein, the receptor-binding domain (RBD) could elicit higher titers of IgG antibodies in mice. Some research showed that RBD-based SARS-CoV subunit vaccines were more effective and safer than other viral vector-based vaccines. It was reported that RBD vaccines administered through intramuscular injections could induce long-term protection against SARS-CoV infections. Thus, targeting the RBD of SARS-CoV-2 is also one of the strategies in vaccine development. As with MERS-CoV, MERS-CoV S377-588-Fc had stronger immunogenicity than the other MERS-CoV RBDs (S367-388-Fc, S358-588-Fc, and S367-606-Fc) and induced significantly higher titers of neutralizing antibodies in vaccinated mice. These antibodies could block the binding of MERS-CoV RBD to the receptor. Two currently available antibodies (REGN3051 and REGN3048) could bind to the RBD of the S protein and inhibit its interaction with dipeptidyl peptidase-4 (DPP4). These antibodies were tested in a mouse model and were effective in inhibiting MERS-CoV replication. However, further testing of these vaccine candidates needs to be conducted in dromedary models.

In addition, it was reported that a humanized monoclonal antibody (mAb YS110) against DPP4 was confirmed to inhibit MERS-CoV infections. Another study revealed that both mice and rabbits developed high titers of neutralizing antibodies when stimulated with MERS-CoV 377-588-Fc. Intranasal inoculation of a MERS-CoV

RBD-based subunit vaccine had great potential to induce a mucosal IgA response against the RBD and MERS-CoV S proteins. However, since the receptor of SARS-CoV-2 is not DPP4, mAb YS110 is not expected to inhibit SARS-CoV-2 infection. Still, this approach of designing a humanized monoclonal antibody against the receptor is worth considering.

7.1.3 *Adjuvant vaccine*

Using vaccines in combination with adjuvants can increase the production of neutralizing antibodies against coronaviruses. It was reported that the inoculation of mice with MERS-CoV S protein alone was not sufficient to induce antibody production; rather, the viral protein bound to an adjuvant could elicit a potent response of neutralizing antibodies. Both potassium aluminum sulfate (alum) and MF59 adjuvants could elicit antigen-specific antibodies and cellular-mediated responses and might be used for MERS-CoV subunit vaccine administration. However, only when combined with another adjuvant (such as a synthetic TLR4 agonist) could alum induce a potent Th1 cellular response. This cocktail could improve the efficacy of the MERS-CoV RBD-based subunit vaccines. Research done by Coleman *et al.* showed that the immune responses to SARS-CoV and MERS-CoV-S could be boosted approximately 15- and 7-fold by using the adjuvants alum and MF59, respectively. Additionally, the use of adjuvants could enhance immunogenicity and safety of MERS-CoV vaccines.

7.2 Research and Development of Vaccines against SARS-CoV-2

Compared to DNA vaccines, mRNA vaccines are a relatively safer type of novel nucleic acid-based vaccines. The sequence design and chemical modification of mRNA vaccines now mainly focus on strengthening their stability and weakening their immunogenicity. As the main molecule in the vaccine, an mRNA has the following advantages over DNA: it does not require any nuclear localization signal (NLS) or transcription, and it is not possible to be integrated into the genome, thus avoiding any unwanted mutation by the vaccination. Moderna, Inc. has been designing an mRNA vaccine against SARS-CoV-2. On February 24, 2020, the company announced that it had completed the development of this vaccine and had shipped the first batch of vaccines to the US National Institutes of Health (NIH) for phase I clinical trial.

On February 25, 2020, Tianjin University announced an oral vaccine against SARS-CoV-2 in development. This novel preparation uses food-grade brewer's yeast (*Saccharomyces cerevisiae*) as a vector and could elicit antibodies against SARS-CoV-2 S protein. Brewer's yeast has long been used as a vaccine vector: its genome sequence is well known; it inherently carries some natural adjuvants and has high safety; it is capable of multiplying rapidly within a short time; and it can be quickly mass produced to meet demands. Thus, utilizing the brewer's yeast offers a new pathway to the development of SARS-CoV-2 vaccines. Thus far, the core techniques relevant to mass-producing the yeast recombinant vaccine have been developed, including construction and screening of the recombinant strain, protein expression, and fermentation kinetics. The subsequent vaccine efficacy and safety trials are currently underway.

7.3 Animal Models

Currently, most research on SARS-CoV-2 vaccines has predicted possible antigen epitopes by means of immunoinformatics or other methodology, rather than testing the vaccines in animal models. In the latest study, researchers successfully constructed an hACE2 transgenic mouse strain by microinjecting the mouse hACE2 promoter into C57BL/6J blastocyst. The transgenic mice were subsequently infected with SARS-CoV-2 to study the pathogenicity of the virus. As one of the latest studies on SARS-CoV-2 animal models, it is very instructive for evaluating the safety and efficacy of SARS-CoV-2 vaccines. We can further refer to past research on SARS-CoV- and MERS-CoV-related vaccines to adopt appropriate animal models for evaluating the safety and protective efficacy of future vaccines against SARS-CoV-2.

7.3.1 *Mouse models*

The mouse strains selected as the animal models for SARS-CoV infection include BALB/c, C57BL/6 (B6), and 129/SvEv. A study used 4- to 8-week-old BALB/c or B6 mice with intranasally inoculated SARS-CoV to gain high titers of viral replication in the lungs. The peak of the viral replication in the respiratory tract was noted two to three days after the infection, without substantial accompanying lung inflammation. Five to seven days after the infection, viruses in the lungs were completely cleared, and protective neutralizing antibodies were seen in mice with sublethal infection. This could possibly reflect the immune status of the infected patients during the SARS epidemic. Thus, mice can be used as stable and replicable models to evaluate the protective efficacy and safety of SARS-CoV vaccines.

Rodents are not susceptible to MERS-CoV infection, primarily because their DPP4 does not function as the receptor for MERS-CoV to mediate viral entry. To date, researchers have developed several mouse models susceptible to MERS-CoV infection. In 2014, it was reported for the first time that the recombinant vaccine based on adenovirus type 5 (Ad5) encoding human DPP4 (hDPP4) was administered to mice through nasal inoculation. MERS-CoV was used to infect the mice so that the virus could replicate in the lungs. The mice then exhibited symptoms of interstitial pneumonia. However, as it is hard to control the expression of hDPP4, this model also has its limitations.

7.3.2 *Hamster models*

Studies showed that Golden Syrian hamsters (*Mesocricetus auratus*) and Chinese hamsters (*Cricetulus griseus*) were also excellent animal models for SARS-CoV infection. Similar to the mouse model, infected hamsters also produce SARS-CoV-specific protective antibodies. As infecting hamsters with SARS-CoV elicits high titers of viral replication and replicable pulmonary pathological lesions, they provide ideal models for studying the immunity to SARS-CoV and prevention from related diseases. However, for hamsters, there is yet to be any genetic-based line with accurate immunological and biological markers, so the use of hamster models will have limitations to some extent.

7.3.3 *Ferret models*

Ferrets (*Mustela putorius furo*) can transmit SARS at low levels by direct contact and exhibit symptoms of fever when infected; these are typical symptoms of patients infected with SARS-CoV, which distinguish ferrets from other animal models. The mortality rate in infected ferrets is not high, making them stable animal models for SARS-CoV infection. However, thus far, there have been inconsistent or even contradictory reports on their histopathological lesions and the severity of clinical symptoms. Further research is necessary.

7.3.4 *Dromedary models*

Dromedaries (*Camelus dromedarius*) are an important host of MERS-CoV. In dromedaries infected with MERS-CoV, viral replication is seen primarily in their upper respiratory tracts. Therefore, researchers may vaccinate intranasally using a mucosal atomization device. However, due to the large size and high cost of the animal, it is hard to conduct large-scale studies on MERS-CoV infections in dromedaries.

7.3.5 *Nonhuman primate models*

To date, there have been six nonhuman primate species evaluated as models of SARS-CoV infection: Rhesus macaque (*Macaca mulatta*), cynomolgus macaque (*Macaca fascicularis*), African green monkey (*Chlorocebus aethiops*), common marmoset (*Callithrix jacchus*), squirrel monkey (*Saimiri sp.*), and mustached tamarin (*Saguinus mystax*). Rhesus macaque and common marmoset are two effective models for research on mild MERS-CoV infection pathogenesis and therapeutic efficacy evaluation.

7.4 Summary and Outlook

Entering the 21st century, we have already seen three large outbreaks of pneumonia caused by coronavirus infections. Each outbreak has taken a heavy toll on the economy and public health, but there is no effective and widely applicable vaccine to date. There has been research showing peaks in the number of patent applications related to human coronavirus vaccines, both globally and domestically in China, that highly coincides with the outbreaks. This also suggests that most research institutions followed the trend of research only to respond to the immediate epidemics, instead of forming a desirable, sustainable research and development strategy. The difficulties in developing coronavirus vaccines may be relevant to the high mutation rate of the viruses and the strict biosafety protocols that it entails. Thus far, there has been research that proposed or predicted the potential targets of vaccines against SARS-CoV-2, but none of them has been tested on animal models for their efficacy and safety. There is still a large gap to be filled in the SARS-CoV-2 vaccine research. The development of vaccines carries great significance in eradicating SARS-CoV-2, preventing the next outbreak of a coronavirus, and easing public concerns.

References

1. Hu HZ, Shen YQ. Novel research progress of the recombinant vaccine for MERS-CoV. [Chinese]. *Chin J Virol.* 2016;495–500:32(04).
2. Xie HL, Lv LC, Yang YP. Patent analysis of global coronavirus vaccines. [Chinese]. *China Biotechnol.* 2020;1–14 [2020-03-18]. http://kns.cnki.net/kcms/detail/11.4816.Q.20200221.1853.002.html.
3. Abdelmageed M, Abdelmoneim AH, Mustafa MI, *et al.* Design of multi epitope-based peptide vaccine against E protein of human 2019-nCoV: An immunoinformatics approach. *bioRxiv.* (2020-02-04) [2020-02-23]. https://doi.org/10.1101/2020.02.04.934232.
4. Chai XQ, Hu LF, Zhang Y, *et al.* Specific ACE2 expression in cholangiocytes may cause liver damage after 2019-nCoV infection. *bioRxiv.* (2020-02-03) [2020-02-23]. https://doi.org/10.1101/2020.02.03.931766.
5. Diao B, Wang C, Tan Y, *et al.* Reduction and functional exhaustion of T cells in patients with coronavirus disease 2019 (COVID-19). *medRxiv.* (2020-02-18) [2020-02-23]. https://doi.org/10.1101/2020.02.18.20024364.
6. Du L, He Y, Zhou Y, *et al.* The spike protein of SARS-CoV — a target for vaccine and therapeutic development. *Nat Rev Microbiol.* 2009;7(3):226–36.

7. Fan CB, Li K, Ding YH, *et al.* ACE2 expression in kidney and testis may cause kidney and testis damage after 2019-nCoV infection. *medRxiv.* (2020-02-12) [2020-02-23]. https://doi.org/10.1101/2020.02.12.20022418.

8. Haagmans BL, van den Brand JM, Raj VS, *et al.* An orthopoxvirus-based vaccine reduces virus excretion after MERS-CoV infection in dromedary camels. *Science.* 2016;351(6268):77–81.

9. Lan J, Ge JW, Yu JF, *et al.* Crystal structure of the 2019-nCoV spike receptor-binding domain bound with the ACE2 receptor. *bioRxiv.* (2020-02-19) [2020-02-23]. https://doi.org/10.1101/2020.02.19.956235.

10. Lei C, Fu W, Qian K, *et al.* Potent neutralization of 2019 novel coronavirus by recombinant ACE2-Ig. *bioRxiv.* (2020-01-29) [2020-02-23]. https://doi.org/10.1101/2020.02.01.929976.

11. Meng T, Cao H, Zhang H, *et al.* The insert sequence in SARS-CoV-2 enhances spike protein cleavage by TMPRSS. *bioRxiv.* (2020-02-08) [2020-02-23]. https://doi.org/10.1101/2020.02.08.926006.

12. Mubarak A, Alturaiki W, Hemida MG. Middle east respiratory syndrome coronavirus (MERS-CoV): Infection, immunological response, and vaccine development. *J Immunol Res.* 2019;1:1–11.

13. Qiu TY, Mao TT, Wang Y, *et al.* Identification of potential cross-protective epitope between 2019-nCoV and SARS virus. *J Genet Genomics.* (2020-01-26) [2020-02-23]. https://doi:10.1016/j.jgg.2020.01.003.

14. Ramaiah A, Arumugaswami V. Insights into cross-species evolution of novel human coronavirus 2019-nCoV and defining immune determinants for vaccine development. *bioRxiv.* (2020-01-29) [2020-02-23]. https://doi.org/10.1101/2020.01.29.925867.

15. Sarkar B, Ullah MA, Johora FT, *et al.* The essential facts of Wuhan Novel Coronavirus outbreak in China and epitope-based vaccine designing against 2019-nCoV. *bioRxiv.* (2020-02-05) [2020-02-23]. https://doi.org/10.1101/2020.02.05.935072.

16. Song Z, Xu Y, Bao L, *et al.* From SARS to MERS, thrusting coronaviruses into the spotlight. *Viruses.* 2019;11(1):59.

17. Tian X, Li C, Huang A, *et al.* Potent binding of 2019 novel coronavirus spike protein by a SARS coronavirus-specific human monoclonal antibody. *bioRxiv.* (2020-01-28) [2020-02-23]. https://doi.org/10.1101/2020.01.28.923011.

18. Xia S, Zhu Y, Liu M, *et al.* Fusion mechanism of 2019-nCoV and fusion inhibitors targeting HR1 domain in spike protein. *Cell Mol Immunol.* (2020-02-11) [2020-02-23]. http://doi.org/10.1038/s41423-020-0374-2.

19. Yan RH, Zhang YY, Guo YY, *et al.* Structural basis for the recognition of the 2019-nCoV by human ACE2. *bioRxiv.* (2020-02-19) [2020-02-23]. https://doi.org/10.1101/2020.02.29.956946.
20. Zou X, Chen K, Zou JW, *et al.* The single-cell RNA-seq data analysis on the receptor ACE2 expression reveals the potential risk of different human organs vulnerable to Wuhan 2019-nCoV infection. *Front Med.* (2020-02-08) [2020-02-23]. https://doi.org/10.1007/s11684-020-0754-0.

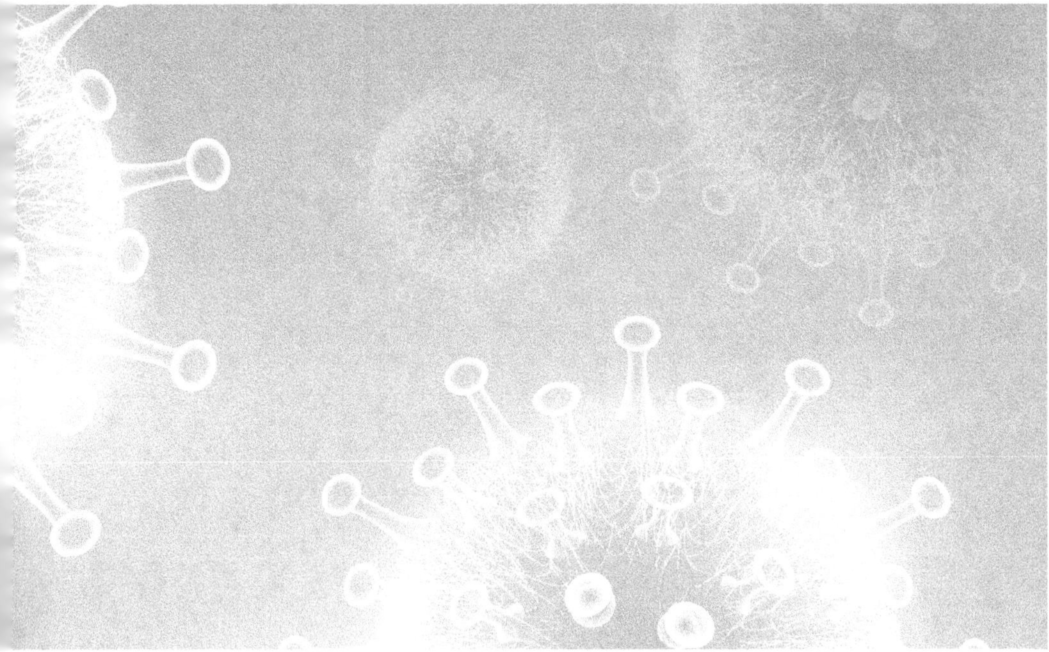

Part 4

Clinical Characteristics

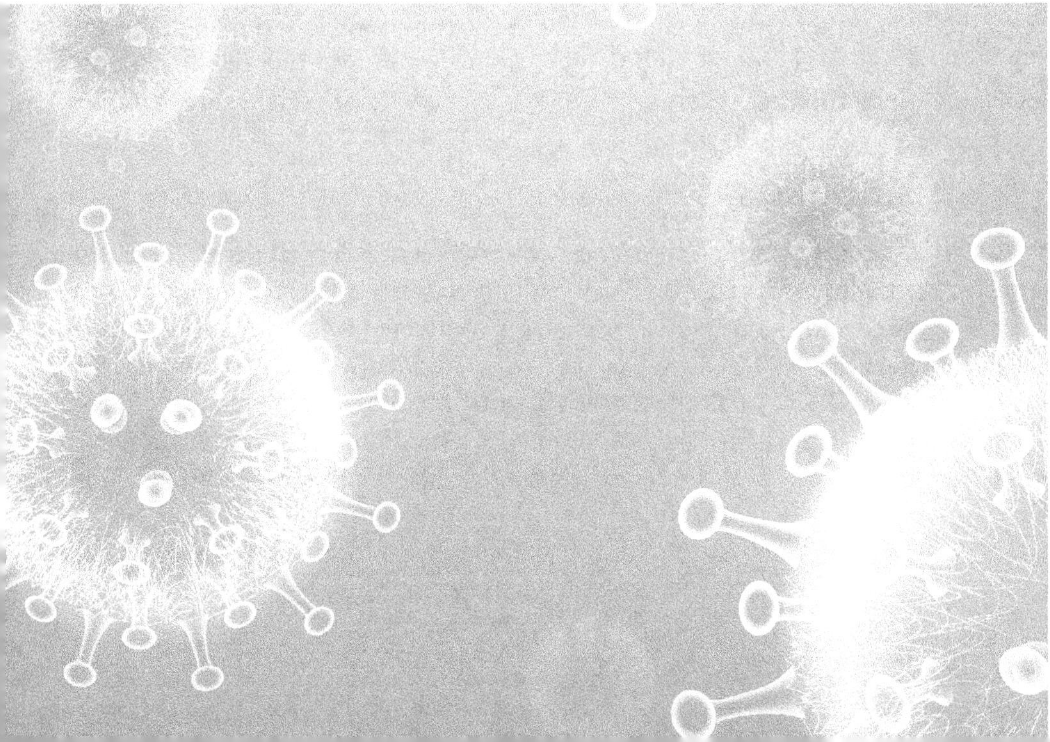

Chapter 8
Clinical Manifestations

8.1 Incubation Period

Based on the epidemiology studies to date, COVID-19 has an incubation period of 1 to 14 days, most frequently 3 to 7 days.

8.2 Clinical Manifestations

The major clinical manifestations of COVID-19 were concluded from retrospective analyses (Table 8-1) of confirmed cases (including patients with severe and non-severe COVID-19 from both Wuhan and other areas in China). The most common clinical manifestations were fever, cough, and fatigue, occurring in over half of the patients on average.

8.2.1 *Systemic symptoms*

The most common systemic symptom was fever, which occurred in over 83% of the COVID-19 patients to various degrees. According to two reports on multilayer analyses conducted on patients; body temperatures, 38.1–39°C was the most frequently seen, accounting for around 45% of all the febrile patients. Majority of patients had disease onset with a fever, mostly a low or a medium fever, and those with continuous high fevers experienced worse conditions. However, it is

Table 8-1. Comparison of clinical manifestations in various retrospective analyses of reported COVID-19 cases

Source	Three hospitals in Beijing	Wuhan Jinyintan Hospital	Zhongnan Hospital of Wuhan University	Other hospitals in Wuhan	From 552 hospitals in other areas of the country
Number of cases	13 cases	99 cases	138 cases	41 cases	1,099 cases
Gender and age	Male: 77% Median age: 34 yrs	Male: 68% Average age: 55.5 yrs	Male: 54.3% Median age: 56 yrs	Male: 73% Median age: 49 yrs	Male: 58.1% Median age: 47 yrs
Subgroups			ICU: 102 cases Non-ICU: 36 cases	ICU: 13 cases Non-ICU: 28 cases	Severe: 173 cases Non-severe: 926 cases
Fever (%)	92.3	83	98.6	98[a]	88.7[b]
Fatigue (%)			69.6	44[c]	38.1
Myalgia (%)	23.1	11	34.8	44[c]	14.9
Headache (%)	23.1	8	6.5	8	13.6
Cough (%)	46.2	82	86.2	76	67.8
Dry cough (%)			59.4		
Sputum production (%)	15.4		26.8	28	33.7
Shortness of breath (%)		31			18.7[d]

[a]The body temperatures of febrile patients most commonly fell in 38.1–39°C (44%).
[b]The body temperatures of febrile patients most commonly fell in 38.1–39°C (46.9%).
[c]Fatigue or myalgia.
[d]Shortness of breath was more common in severe patients (37.6% *vs.* 15.1%, $P < 0.001$).

Table 8.1.   (*Continued*)

Source	Three hospitals in Beijing	Wuhan Jinyintan Hospital	Zhongnan Hospital of Wuhan University	Other hospitals in Wuhan	From 552 hospitals in other areas of the country
Dyspnea (%)			31.2[f]	55[e]	
Sore throat (%)		5	17.4[g]		13.9
Rhinorrhea (%)	7.7	4			
Nausea/Emesis (%)		Both occurring: 1	Nausea: 10.1 Vomiting: 3.6		Nausea or vomiting: 5
Diarrhea (%)	7.7	2	10.1	3	3.8
Other symptoms (%)		Chest pain: 2	Abdominal pain: 2.2 Loss of appetite: 39.9	Hemoptysis: 5	Nasal congestion: 4.8 Chills: 11.5

[e]Dyspnea was more common in ICU patients (92% *vs.* 37%, $P = 0.001$). The median time from disease onset to dyspnea was 8 days (IQR: 5–13 days).

[f]Dyspnea was more common in ICU patients (63.9% *vs.* 19.6%, $P < 0.001$). The median time from disease onset to dyspnea was 5 days (IQR: 1–10 days).

[g]Sore throat was more common in ICU patients (33.3% *vs.* 11.8%, $P = 0.003$).

worth noting that some of the patients with severe COVID-19 had low or medium fevers, or even no fever. Fatigue was also one of the most common nonspecific symptoms, observed in 38–70% of the patients. In addition, myalgia was also a nonspecific symptom brought to attention in many studies, having been observed in 10–45% of the cases. In *Diagnosis and Treatment Protocol for COVID-19 (6th trial version)*, myalgia was listed as one of the clinical manifestations. Meanwhile, headache was a relatively less common symptom.

8.2.2 *Respiratory symptoms*

The respiratory tract was the main site attacked by SARS-CoV-2. Among all the respiratory symptoms in COVID-19, cough was the most prevalent. It was observed in over 70% of patients, among which dry cough was more common. Shortness of breath (incidence rate: 18–31%) and dyspnea (incidence rate: 31–55%) were also seen in reports on respiratory symptoms. Subgroup analysis of all the cases showed that shortness of breath and dyspnea were more likely to occur ($P \leq 0.001$) in patients admitted to ICUs, with the median time ranging from 5 to 8 days from disease onset to dyspnea. Therefore, the patients' conditions should be closely monitored within a week from the disease onset, so that the severe cases could be recognized as soon as possible. Respiratory symptoms like sore throat and rhinorrhea were less seen.

8.2.3 *Gastrointestinal symptoms*

Similar to SARS, COVID-19 also affected patients' gastrointestinal tract. The incidence rate of diarrhea was 2–10%, which warrants attention from clinicians. Additionally, nausea and vomiting were relatively less common gastrointestinal symptoms.

8.2.4 *Other rare clinical manifestations*

Some retrospective studies showed other rarely seen and not commonly reported clinical manifestations, including but not limited to hemoptysis, chest pain, abdominal pain, and chill. Such manifestations are not elaborated here.

8.2.5 *Asymptomatic infections*

As the epidemic developed, asymptomatic cases were occasionally found in various places; these patients were contagious to some extent. The statement that "asymptomatic infected cases might also become sources of infection" had been added to the epidemiological characteristics since the 5th trial version of the *Diagnosis and Treatment Protocol for COVID-19* in China. A typical case was that a female patient from Wuhan going back to Anyang, Henan province had caused five close contacts to be diagnosed with COVID-19 while experiencing no symptoms. *The New England Journal of Medicine* also reported that among the 126 German citizens evacuated from Wuhan to Germany, one had no symptoms but tested positive for the SARS-CoV-2 RNA. However, it is still too early to conclude whether the asymptomatic cases found so far were indeed "asymptomatic", or they were presymptomatic and still in the incubation period, or their symptoms were too mild to be felt. In future, retrospective serological research is necessary to further elucidate the actual incidence rate of asymptomatic COVID-19 infection in the population and its epidemiological significance.

8.3 Clinical Classification

According to China;s *Diagnosis and Treatment Protocol for Novel Coronavirus Pneumonia (6th trial version)*, COVID-19 cases can be categorized into four clinical types: mild cases, moderate cases, severe cases, and critical cases.

(1) Mild cases exhibit mild symptoms including low fever and mild fatigue, with no sign of pneumonia in chest imaging. Mild cases made up approximately 5% of all cases. Clinicians should note, however, that patients thus classified at the early stage of their disease onset might have conditions that progress further.

(2) Moderate cases exhibit fever and respiratory symptoms, with chest imaging showing features of pneumonia. It was the most common type of COVID-19 cases, accounting for approximately 80% of all cases.

(3) Cases meeting any of the following criteria should be considered a severe case: (1) shortness of breath, RR (respiratory rate) $\geq$ 30 breaths/min; (2) pulse oxygen saturation $\leq$ 93% at rest; (3) arterial oxygen partial pressure $(PaPO_2)$/fraction of inspiration oxygen (FiO_2) $\leq$ 300 mmHg (1 mmHg = 0.133kPa), where in high-altitude areas (over 1,000 m above sea level), PaO_2/FiO_2 should be corrected using the following formula: $PaO_2/FiO_2 \times$ [atmospheric pressure (mmHg)/760]; and (4) chest imaging showing obvious lesion progression >50% within 24–48 hours.

(4) If the disease progresses and any of the following conditions are observed, it should be considered a critical case: (1) respiratory failure and mechanical ventilation required; (2) shock; and (3) combination with other organ failure with intensive care in ICU needed. It is worth noting that severe and critical cases could exhibit low or medium fevers, or even no observable fever along the course of the disease.

Chapter 9
Chest Imaging

Chest imaging plays a vital role in COVID-19 screening, early diagnosis, disease evaluation, and follow-up. Since little abnormality could be observed on chest radiographs at the early stage of the disease because of its low sensitivity, we recommend lung computed tomography (CT) screening as the preferred radiology diagnostic method. Mastering the common and typical manifestations of COVID-19 on lung CT scan is important for identifying patients and assessing disease progression.

9.1 Common CT Manifestations

Based on the case reports and summaries to date, the most common findings of COVID-19 seen on lung CT were ground-glass opacity (GGO) and consolidation, usually located in multiple lobes bilaterally and mainly peripherally. The opacification of GGO was slightly increased, which does not obscure the blood vessels and airways, while that of consolidation obscures blood vessels and airway walls. On average, over 80% of the COVID-19 cases presented with pneumonia had lung CT results featuring one of the previously mentioned signs. As summarized in an article, GGOs were already commonly observed on lung CT within the first four days after symptom onset. Subsequently, as the disease progressed, crazy-paving patterns (the thickening of inter- and intralobular septa superimposed on GGO lesions) and consolidation developed; reversed halo signs (mostly a rounded GGO surrounded by a ring of consolidation) could be found on the lung CT in some cases. According to the studies thus far, the chest imaging of COVID-19 had the most extensive manifestations 10–14 days from the symptom onset, on average. Rare CT findings included pleural effusion, thoracic lymphadenopathy, scattered nodular lesions, and cavitation.

9.2 Stages of CT Manifestations

The manifestations of lung CT in COVID-19 are related to the stage of clinical course after infection. According to *Radiologic Diagnosis of New Coronavirus Infected Pneumonitis: Expert Recommendation from the Chinese Society of Radiology* (*First Edition*), the findings of lung CT in COVID-19 can be categorized into the following four stages. There may be overlaps and transitions between the stages.

9.2.1 *Early stage*

The lung CT at this stage manifests single or multiple localized ground-glass opacities (Figure 9-1) — most of which are round — as

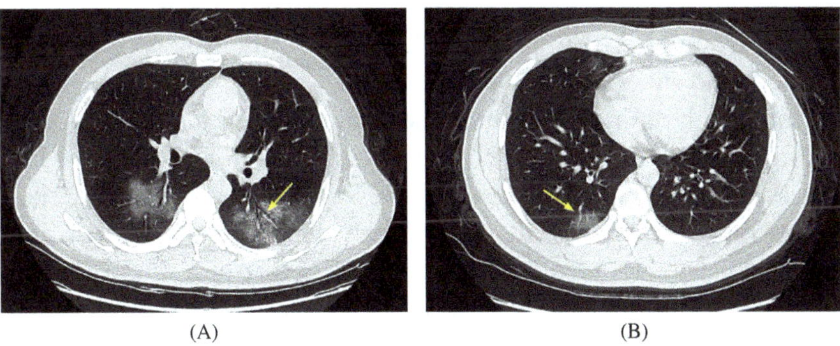

(A)   (B)

Figure 9-1. Lung CT manifestation at the early stage of COVID-19 (1)

A: Male patient, 38 years old, a confirmed case of COVID-19. Lung CT manifested GGO along with bronchovascular bundles, within which the thickened vascular shadows and air bronchogram signs could be seen (arrow). **B**: Male patient, 29 years old, a confirmed case of COVID-19, whose lung CT manifested subpleural GGO, within which the thicken vascular shadows could be seen (arrow).

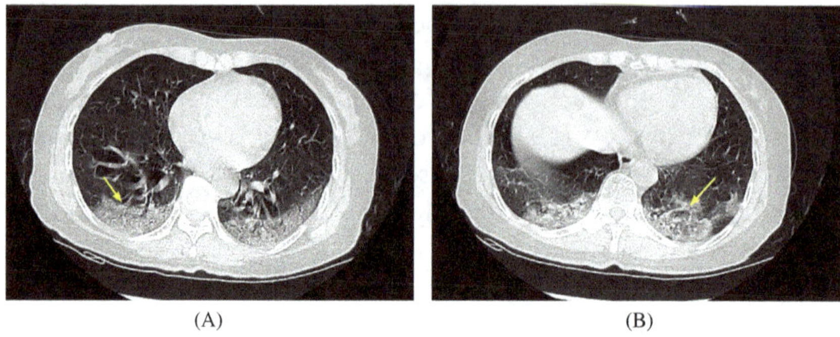

(A)   (B)

Figure 9-2.   Lung CT manifestation at the early stage of COVID-19 (2)

Female patient, 60 years old, a confirmed case of COVID-19. Typical lung CT manifestations relevant to COVID-19. **A**: Bilateral GGO with thin grid-like shadow (arrow). **B**: A reversed halo sign (arrow) in left lower lobe, which was a GGO surrounded by a ring of consolidation.

well as subpleural flakes with their long axes parallel to pleurae. The lesions are usually subpleural or under the interlobar fissure, or along the bronchovascular bundles, mainly in the lower and middle lobes. In GGO lesions, some bronchiolar walls and blood vessels thicken. As the disease progresses, interlobular septa in some GGO lesions thicken and could manifest themselves as thin grid-like shadows or crazy-paving patterns (Figure 9-2A). In addition, consolidation can develop around some other GGO shadows, manifesting themselves as reversed halo signs (Figure 9-2B).

It is worth noting that some articles summarized lung CT findings at different time points, and concluded that within the first two days after symptom onset, more than half (56%) of the analyzed cases had no abnormality on lung CT, while after the first two days, the percentage dropped to less than 10%. This indicates that lung CT can show no apparent abnormality at a very early stage of the disease. Thus, chest imaging alone is not reliable enough to rule out COVID-19.

9.2.2 *Progressive stage*

COVID-19 usually progresses quickly; the lung CT findings at the progressive stage usually manifest an increase on the lesion number,

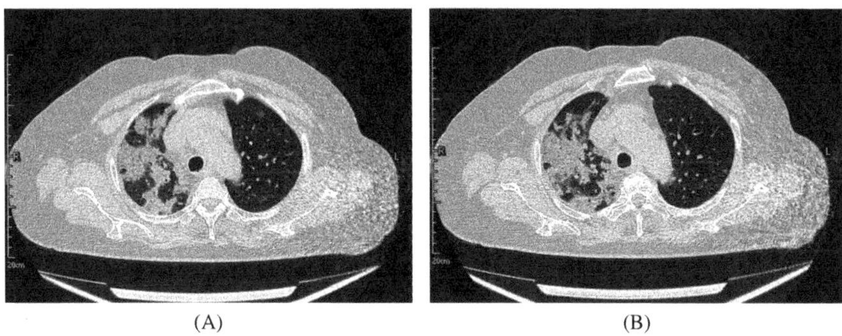

(A)   (B)

Figure 9-3. Lung CT manifestation at the progressive stage of COVID-19

Female patient, 60 years old, a confirmed case of COVID-19. Lung CT manifested multiple consolidations with partial fusion.

the partial fusion of lesions, the enlargement of lesions, and an increase in the lesion density. Consolidations to various degrees also appear, with air bronchogram signs inside (Figure 9-3).

9.2.3 *Severe stage*

As the disease progresses, CT findings become more extensive at the severe stage. Bilateral diffused consolidations (Figure 9-4) with

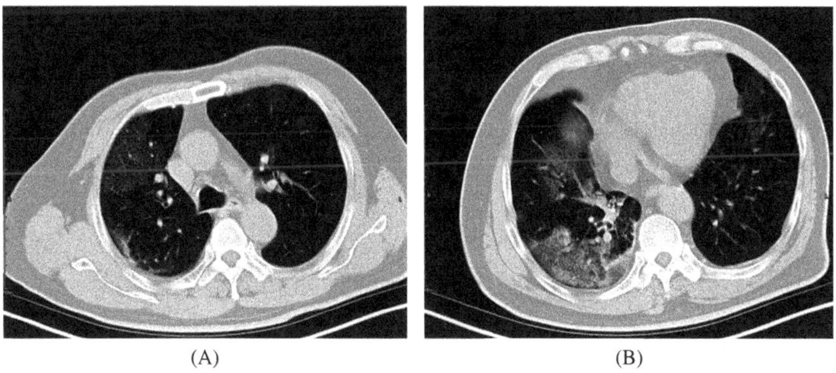

(A)   (B)

Figure 9-4. Lung CT manifestation at the severe stage of COVID-19

Male patient, 64 years old, a confirmed case of COVID-19, with type 2 diabetes. Lung CT manifested multiple GGOs and consolidations bilaterally.

uneven density can be seen, as well as air bronchogram signs inside. In areas without consolidations, patchy GGOs can be seen. When most of the bilateral lungs are affected by the disease, lung CT manifests "white lung" features. Interlobar and pulmonary pleurae usually become thickened. A little pleural effusion can be seen in some cases.

9.2.4 *Recovery stage*

After isolation and treatment, most COVID-19 patients have their conditions stabilized and become better. Lung CT manifestations include gradually absorbed lesions, while cord-like shadows can be left behind in some cases (Figure 9-5). A small number of cases have a rather short course, which can develop from the early stage directly into the recovery stage.

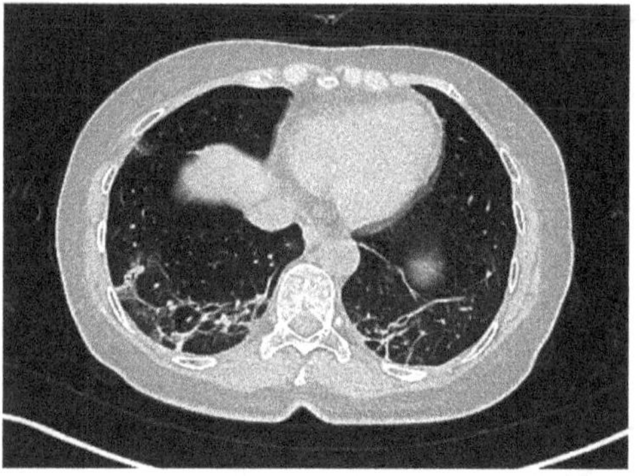

Figure 9-5.   Lung CT manifestation at the recovery stage of COVID-19

Female patient, 60 years old, a confirmed case of COVID-19. After isolation and treatment, her lung CT manifested gradually absorbed lesions, with cord-like shadows being left behind.

9.3 Atypical CT Manifestation

Some atypical or rare COVID-19 chest radiological manifestations were only seen in reports of individual cases, including cord-like shadows, cavitation, halo signs, multiple nodules, etc.

Chapter 10
Laboratory Diagnosis

10.1 Laboratory Test Results

In the early stage of COVID-19, patients often have normal or low white blood cell counts and low lymphocyte counts. These laboratory results, combined with exposure and contact history, fever, respiratory symptoms, and chest imaging, are important features of suspected cases of COVID-19. In addition, many patients have high levels of C-reactive protein (CRP), elevated erythrocyte sedimentation rate (ESR), and normal procalcitonin, while some may have elevated liver enzymes, lactate dehydrogenase (LDH), creatine kinase (CK), and myoglobin (mostly transient). Patients in serious or critical conditions may have significantly increased troponin, D-dimer, and other inflammatory factors, accompanied by progressive reduction of peripheral blood lymphocytes.

10.2 Specimen Types and Collection Methods for Etiology Diagnosis

Suspected cases are confirmed when they meet one of these etiological criteria: (1) Positive SARS-CoV-2 RT-PCR test and (2) viral genome sequence highly homologous to known SARS-CoV-2. Adequate and appropriate specimen collection is very important for COVID-19. Proper collection methods and appropriation location are to be emphasized in specimen collection. Currently acceptable specimens include those from upper and lower respiratory tract, blood, serum, conjunctiva, and stool. At present, according to the "Laboratory Biosafety Guidance for the Novel Coronavirus (nCoV, SARS-CoV-2) (second edition)" and "Laboratory Testing and Biosafety Practices and Procedures for the Novel Coronavirus (nCoV, SARS-CoV-2)", the guidelines for specimen collection are as follows.

10.2.1 *Respiratory tract specimen collection*

Respiratory tract specimens include: throat (oropharyngeal) swab, nasal swab, nasopharyngeal aspirate, deep cough phlegm, respiratory tract aspirate, bronchial lavage, and bronchoalveolar lavage (BAL). The recommended specimen collection methods are as follows:

(1) Throat (oropharyngeal) swab: Use two polyester flocked plastic swabs to swab into both pharyngeal tonsils and the posterior pharynx. Snap the swab shaft off at the score and leave the swab inside the tube with 3 ml virus transport medium (saline or cell culture medium), and tighten the cap securely.

(2) Nasal swab: Gently insert a polypropylene flocked plastic swab into the nasal palate. Keep the swab in place for a few seconds and slowly rotate and withdraw the swab. Take another polypropylene flocked plastic swab to collect from the other nostril in the same way. Snap the swab shafts off at the score and leave the swabs inside the same tube with 3 ml virus transport medium and tighten the cap securely.

(3) Nasopharyngeal aspirate or respiratory tract aspirate: Use a collector fitted to a suction pump to draw samples from the nasopharynx or respiratory tract secretion from the trachea. Insert the collector head into the nasal cavity or trachea. Apply suction and slowly withdraw the collector head with a rotating motion. Collect the mucus and rinse the collector once with 3 ml virus transport medium. (The collector may be replaced by a pediatric catheter connected to a 50 ml syringe.)

(4) Deep cough phlegm: Let the patient expectorate coughed-up phlegm and collect the specimen with a 50 ml screw-cap collection tube containing 3 ml virus transport medium.

(5) Bronchial lavage: Insert the collector head into the trachea (about 30 cm deep) from the nostril or tracheal tube. Inject 5 ml saline. Apply suction, and slowly withdraw the collector head with a rotating motion. Collect the mucus and rinse the collector once with virus transport medium. (The collector may be replaced by a pediatric catheter connected to a 50 ml syringe.)

(6) Bronchoalveolar lavage (BAL): After local anesthesia, insert the fiberoptic bronchoscope from the mouth or nose through the pharynx into the bronchus of the middle lobe of the right lung or the lingula of the left lung, and insert the distal tip into the bronchial branching point. Slowly add sterile saline through the tracheal biopsy channel, 30–50 ml each time. Total volume is 100–250 ml and should not exceed 300 ml.

10.2.2 *Blood specimen collection*

Blood specimens include: whole blood and serum specimens.

(1) Whole blood: Try to collect blood with anticoagulant in the acute phase within seven days after disease onset. Collect 5 ml, preferably fasting blood. It is recommended to use a Vacutainer blood collection tube containing ethylenediaminetetraacetic acid (EDTA) anticoagulant to collect blood. Let the specimen stand at room temperature for 30 minutes and then centrifuge it at 1,500–2,000 r/min for ten minutes.

(2) Serum: Try to collect it in both acute phase and recovery phase. The first serum should be collected as soon as possible (preferably seven to ten days after onset). The second serum should be collected three to four weeks after onset. The collection volume is 5 ml, preferably fasting blood. It is recommended to use an evacuated Vacutainer blood collection tube to collect 5 ml blood. Let the specimen stand at room temperature for 30

minutes and then centrifuge it at 1,500–2,000 r/min for ten minutes.

10.2.3 *Collection of other specimens*

In addition to respiratory specimens and blood specimens, some studies have suggested that viral nucleic acid can be detected in conjunctival specimen and stool specimen.

(1) Conjunctival specimen: In cases with eye infection symptoms, a conjunctival swab needs to be collected. After gently swabbing the conjunctival surface, insert the swab tip into a tube, snap the swab shaft off, and tighten the cap securely.
(2) Stool specimen: For patients with diarrhea symptoms, stool specimen needs to be collected. Collect three to 5 ml stool specimen.

10.3 Testing Laboratory Biosafety Guidelines

Biosafety precautions are very important for authorized laboratories to handle SARS-CoV-2 testing. Transport of specimens should adhere to the following principles.

10.3.1 *Transport in the hospital*

After collecting the specimen in the hospital, the outer surface of the specimen container should be wiped or sprayed with 1000 mg/L chlorine-containing disinfectant. Put the specimen container into a dedicated specimen Ziplock bag with a biohazard warning label. Decontaminate the outer surface of the Ziplock bag with 1000 mg/L chlorine-containing disinfectant. Put the bag into a dedicated sealable specimen transport box. Decontaminate the outer surface of the transport box with 1000 mg/L chlorine-containing disinfectant. Personnel must receive biosafety training to transport the specimen to the laboratory. The transport personnel should use first level personal protective equipment (PPE) (wear a cap, disposable surgical mask, gloves, and isolation gown). Keep the transport box steady and avoid jolts during the transport.

10.3.2 *Transport out of the hospital*

If the specimen needs to be transported out of the hospital, the procedure should follow the "Regulation for the Transport of Infectious and Highly Pathogenic Microorganisms (Virus) Strains or Specimens Affecting Humans" (Ministry of Health of the People's Republic of China Order No. 45). According to the Chinese "Technical Guide of Laboratory Testing for the Novel Coronavirus (nCoV, SARS-CoV-2) Pneumonia (Coronavirus Disease 2019, COVID-19)", the shipment packaging classification for SARS-CoV-2 strains and other potentially infectious substances belongs to Category A. The assigned United Nations number is UN2814 (Infectious Substance Affecting Humans). The packaging should comply with Packing Instruction P620 (PI602 for ICAO/IATA regulations).

10.3.3 *Specimen acceptance*

Laboratory staff should decontaminate the transport box with 1000 mg/L chlorine-containing disinfectant before opening. Then decontaminate the Ziplock bag with 1000 mg/L chlorine-containing disinfectant. Open the Ziplock bag in a biosafety cabinet (BSC). Take out the specimen and check specimen information in detail. Register the specimen transfer.

10.3.4 *Laboratory practice and environmental disinfection*

Staff should work in a Biosafety Level 3 (BSL3) laboratory and always operate in a biosafety cabinet (BSC). The laboratory should be equipped with sufficient air sterilizers and/or ultraviolet (UV) lamps. Routine sterilization should be done daily before and after testing (air sterilizer 1 hour each time, UV lamp 30–60 minutes each time). At the same time, 1000 mg/L chlorine-containing disinfectant should be used daily to decontaminate desktops, countertops, floors, door handles, and other touchpoints and surfaces before and after testing. The containers for specimen transport and storage should be wiped with 1000 mg/L chlorine-containing disinfectant before and after use.

10.4 RT-PCR Test

10.4.1 *Introduction of RT-PCR test method*

RT-PCR (reverse-transcription polymerase chain reaction) is currently the most commonly used molecular diagnostic test in clinical practice. A suspected case with positive RT-PCR test result would lead to confirmed diagnosis. If RT-PCR test results are negative in two consecutive tests (specimens collected at least 1 day apart), combined with the patient's clinical symptoms and chest imaging changes, the patient could discontinue isolation and/or be discharged.

At present, many companies in China and abroad have developed and produced RT-PCR test kits for SARS-CoV-2 viral nucleic acid tests. The typical β-coronavirus genome consists of 5′ untranslated region (UTR), *ORF1ab*, *S* gene, *E* gene, *M* gene, *N* gene, 3′UTR, and some unidentified and nonstructural open reading frames (ORF). The current nucleic acid amplification test method mainly targets open reading frames (ORF) of *ORF1ab*, *S*, *E*, *M*, and *N* genes. At present, test kits on the market target either one, two, or three genes. Current research shows that the *ORF1ab* and *S* gene are species specific, and can effectively distinguish SARS-CoV-2 from other coronaviruses (including SARS-CoV), while the *N* and *E* genes in SARS-CoV-2 may cross-react with other coronaviruses (have cross-species amplification and detection in test when other coronaviruses are present). More research is still needed to explore the optimal nucleic acid amplification target combination of SARS-CoV-2.

10.4.2 *Recommended primers and probes and result interpretation*

(1) SARS-CoV-2 nucleic acid detection (by RT-PCR): It is recommended to select primers and probes targeted at the *ORF1ab* and *N* gene of SARS-CoV-2 (Table 10-1).

Table 10-1. Primer and probe sequences recommended for RT-PCR detection by the National Health Commission of the People's Republic of China

Target		Sequence
Target 1 (*ORF1ab*)	Forward primer	5′ — CCCTGTGGGTTTTACACTTAA — 3′
	Reverse primer	5′ — ACGATTGTGCATCAGCTGA — 3′
	Fluorescent probe	5′ — FAM — CCGTCTGCGGTATGTGGAAAGGTTAT-GG — BHQ1 — 3′
Target 2 (*N*)	Forward primer	5′ — GGGGAACTTCTCCTGCTAGAAT — 3′
	Reverse primer	5′ — CAGACATTTTGCTCTCAAGCTG — 3′
	Fluorescent probe	5′ — FAM — TTGCTGCTGCTTGACAGATT — TAMRA — 3′

(2) Result interpretation: Negative: No Ct value or Ct value $\geq$ 40. Positive: Ct value < 37. Grey area: Ct value between 37 and 40. When the Ct value is in the grey area, it is recommended to repeat the test. If the retest Ct value < 40, and the amplification curve has obvious peaks, the test result should be reported as positive, otherwise the test result is negative.

10.4.3 *Causes for false negative results in RT-PCR test*

Clinically, it has been reported that patients with nasal and/or throat (oropharyngeal) swabs had tested negative several times for RT-PCR tests before eventually tested positive. There are multiple possibilities for false negatives in RT-PCR tests. First, improper specimen collection may increase the possibility of false negatives. Second, specimen location may also affect the true positive rate (sensitivity). For mild cases of COVID-19, upper respiratory tract specimen may be collected, while bronchoalveolar lavage (BAL) is preferred in serious cases. However, considering the highly infectious nature of the disease, biosafety guidelines must be strictly followed when an invasive procedure is conducted. In addition, the efficiency of RNA extraction, the quality of the test kit, and potential interference of multiple primers in design may also affect the sensitivity of RT-PCR test. If the virus mutates in genomic regions targeted by primers and/or probes (although these regions are mostly conserved sequences), the mutation may also cause false negatives. Other factors that may produce false negatives also need to be excluded, including poor specimen quality, specimen collected too early or too late, improper specimen storage, transport or processing, or technical difficulties and limitation.

In addition to respiratory specimens, multiple studies have reported that viral nucleic acid can be detected in the blood, stool, and conjunctival secretion of some patients. However, the clinical significance and virulence of nucleic acid isolated from these specimens are still unclear and need to be followed up by further investigation.

Therefore, for highly suspected clinical cases, repeating specimen collection, running multiple tests, changing specimen location, and improving detection method may be used to further increase the sensitivity of RT-PCR test.

10.5 Metagenomic Sequencing

Obtaining genomic sequence of SARS-CoV-2 is another molecular diagnostic method. Metagenomic sequencing (including short-read and long-read sequencing) can obtain genome data from known and novel pathogens. The advantages of metagenomic sequencing are its fast speed, high sensitivity, and unbiased nature, which enable it to play a vital role in diagnosing pneumonia of unknown causes, especially when atypical pathogens are encountered. However, the application of metagenomics has limitations. The current bioinformatics pipeline works by mapping the reads of sequencing to reference databases containing known microbial genomes. This method may cause partial alignment between the novel pathogen genome and previously identified microbial genomes, and lead to incorrect taxonomic classification. In fact, at the beginning of the SARS-CoV-2 infection outbreak, the press cited a sequencing report suggesting identification of SARS-CoV, which caused widespread concern in society. It was later found that the pathogen was a different virus only after an in-depth analysis of the sequencing data obtained. Therefore, for metagenomic method, the sequencing results should always be interpreted in consultation with health professionals, especially when dealing with cases caused by possible novel pathogens or clustered cases.

RNA extraction efficiency, reverse transcription efficiency, sequencing data volume, and bioinformatic analysis are all the factors that may affect the sensitivity of metagenomic method, though still satisfactory compared with that of RT-PCR. In addition, the unbiased sequencing may provide higher sensitivity for detection of genetic variation in target pathogens. Combined with targeted metagenomic sequencing, it enables close monitoring of the molecular evolution of SARS-CoV-2, and provides valuable insights for public health management.

10.6 Serological Test

Compared with RT-PCR and metagenomic sequencing, serological test is faster and more convenient. However, the sensitivity and specificity of serological test may be slightly lower, and needs to be combined with other diagnostic methods. Serological test may detect antigens, immunoglobin M (IgM), IgG, etc. At present, various antibody test kits have been developed in China and abroad. The window period for the appearance of antigens, IgM, and IgG still needs to be further explored for us to understand the best value of serological test.

10.7 Viral Culture *In Vitro*

In vitro culture is a classic method to isolate and obtain viruses. When isolated and cultured *in vitro*, SARS-CoV-2 can be found in human respiratory epithelial cells in about 96 hours, while it took about six days in Vero E6 (African green monkey kidney) cell and Huh-7 (human hepatocellular carcinoma) cell. However, *in vitro* culture of SARS-CoV-2 needs to be carried out in a Biosafety Level 3 (BSL3) laboratory and consumes much time. Thus, it is not recommended as a routine diagnostic method.

10.8 Other Detection Methods

For SARS-CoV-2 detection, fully automated molecular diagnostic system and bedside point-of-care testing (POCT) are also worth exploring. The former can reduce the contamination rate in laboratory operation, while the latter can speed up patient screening. Other detection methods such as loop-mediated isothermal amplification (LAMP) and CRISPR (clustered regularly interspaced short palindromic repeats) may also play a role in SARS-CoV-2 detection.

10.9 Pathogen Detection for Pneumonia of Unknown Causes

It should be noted that there are many infectious respiratory diseases prevalent in winter, which may be caused by influenza viruses, non-SARS-CoV-2 coronaviruses, respiratory syncytial virus (RSV), etc. For patients with pneumonia of unknown causes, clinicians should make a differential diagnosis for other pathogens, and those with testing capacities should screen for other pathogens simultaneously. At present, many studies have found that SARS-CoV-2 co-infects with other viruses. Therefore, during the outbreak, tests for influenza A virus, influenza B virus, RSV, adenovirus, and other pathogens should also be included for the diagnosis of unexplained pneumonia. Clinicians should fully consider the pros and cons of each diagnostic test and use it appropriately to obtain more information for an accurate clinical diagnosis.

Chapter 11
Pathology

COVID-19 is an emerging infectious disease. At present, the understanding of its pathogenesis, pathological features, histological damage, etc. is still based on the previous research on severe acute respiratory syndrome (SARS) and Middle East respiratory syndrome (MERS), and demands further research. Pathological anatomy is essential to answer these questions.

The world's first COVID-19 patient pathology report was completed by postmortem minimally invasive biopsies and was published on *The Lancet Respiratory Medicine*. The study was conducted by a team led by Professors Zhao Jingmin and Wang Fusheng in the Fifth Medical Center of People's Liberation Army General Hospital. Specimens were taken from lung, liver, and heart tissue of the patient. Histological examination revealed bilateral diffuse alveolar damage with cellular fibromyxoid exudates. The right lung displayed evident pneumocyte desquamation and hyaline membrane formation, indicating acute respiratory distress syndrome (ARDS). The left lung tissue showed pulmonary edema with hyaline membrane formation, suggesting early phase ARDS. Interstitial mononuclear inflammatory infiltrates, dominated by lymphocytes, were seen in both lungs. Multinucleated giant cells (MGC), and atypical enlarged pneumocytes characterized by large nuclei, amphophilic granular cytoplasm, and prominent nucleoli were identified in the intra-alveolar spaces, showing viral cytopathic effect. The patient's liver biopsy specimens showed moderate microvesicular steatosis and mild lobular and portal activity; the injury may have been caused by either viral infection or drug-induced liver injury. There were a few interstitial mononuclear inflammatory infiltrates in the heart tissue. The pathology report indicates that the pathological features of SARS-CoV-2 infection greatly resemble those seen in SARS and MERS. The report suggests that SARS-CoV-2 infection mainly affects the lungs and causes severe lung damage; SARS-CoV-2 might not directly attack the liver and heart.

Another paper in preprint first reported clinical pathology of a critical patient with COVID-19, including microscopy, immunohistochemistry, and special staining. The report was completed by Chinese National Research Center for Infectious Diseases and Shenzhen Third People's Hospital (The Second Affiliated Hospital of Southern University of Science and Technology). The study was completed by postmortem lung organ dissection of a COVID-19 patient, and subsequent hematoxylin and eosin staining (HE staining), immunohistochemistry, and special staining including Masson staining, periodic acid-Schiff staining (PAS staining), and methenamine silver staining. The study found that the entire lung tissue showed diffuse congestion or partial hemorrhagic necrosis on gross examination. The hemorrhagic necrosis was prominent on the edge of the lobes of the right lung. The cut surfaces of the lung showed severe congestive and hemorrhagic changes. The main pathological changes of the lung under microscope showed bronchiolitis and alveolitis with proliferation, atrophy, desquamation, and squamous metaplasia of epithelial cells. There were massive pulmonary interstitial fibrosis, partly hyaline degeneration, and various degrees of hemorrhagic pulmonary infarction.There were also small vessel hyperplasia, vessel wall thickening, lumen stenosis, occlusion, and microthrombosis formation. Focal monocytes, lymphocytes, and plasma cells infiltrated into pulmonary interstitium. Atrophy, vacuolar degeneration, proliferation, desquamation, and squamous metaplasia occurred in alveolar epithelial cells. Alveolar congestion was prominent, and contained mucus, edema fluid, desquamated epithelial cells, and inflammatory cells. The study also found some MGC and intracytoplasmic viral inclusion bodies under the microscope. Masson staining indicated massive pulmonary interstitial fibrosis. Immunohistochemical results showed positive for immune cells with leukocyte differentiation antigen (cluster of differentiation, CD) CD3, CD4, CD8, CD20, CD79a, CD5, CD38, and CD68. The study provides solid evidence for the pathogenesis of COVID-19 in critical patients.

In short, there are currently a limited number of publications on the pathological changes of COVID-19 in the world, which only reveals the pathological changes of a few patients at a certain stage of disease development, and cannot fully reflect the pathological damage caused by COVID-19. The overall pathological changes of COVID-19 need to be further studied.

Chapter 12
Prognosis and Outcome

To some extent, COVID-19 is a self-limiting disease with most mild or moderate cases having a favorable prognosis and a course of disease ranging from two to four weeks. Death cases are more common in the elderly and those with chronic underlying conditions.

It was reported that 20–25% of cases developed into severe and critical cases with poor prognosis, among which elderly men were the most common. According to large-scale investigation on the early outbreak of COVID-19 in China, the crude case-fatality rate was estimated at 2–3% and the density was 0.015 per ten person-days, which means the average risk of death for each patient during a 10-day observation was 0.015. The age group of over 80 had the highest crude case-fatality rate of 14.8%. Men had a 2.8% crude case-fatality rate, slightly higher than that of women (1.7%). Hubei province had a 2.9% crude case-fatality rate, which was significantly higher than that of other provinces in China (0.4%). Patients with no reported comorbidities had a 0.9% crude case-fatality rate while the fatality rate was elevated among those with comorbidities — 10.5% for cardiovascular disease, 7.3% for diabetes, 6.3% for chronic respiratory diseases, 6.0% for hypertension, and 5.6% for cancer. Once developed into critical cases, the fatality rate increased significantly. According to previous studies, critical cases had a 49% crude case-fatality rate with a density of 0.325, which means the average risk of death for each critical case during a 10-day observation is 0.325. According to the World Health Organization (WHO), the crude case-fatality rate outside Mainland China was approximately 0.3% (as of February 20, 2020), which was close to that of other provinces and cities outside Hubei in China.

However, current fatality rate estimates rely on limited data of the typical time intervals from symptom onset to death or recovery, and might not accurately reflect the severity of the disease. The published analyses indicated that besides the aforementioned advanced age, comorbidities, and other factors, the prognosis was also related to decreased lymphocyte count and severity of the chest CT lesion. Symptoms in children were relatively mild.

References

1. Bernheim A, Mei X, Huang M, *et al.* Chest CT findings in coronavirus disease-19 (COVID-19): Relationship to duration of infection. *Radiol.* February 2020. http://pubs.rsna.org/doi/10.1148/radiol.2020200463.
2. Chan J F-W, Yuan S, Kok K-H, *et al.* A familial cluster of pneumonia associated with the 2019 novel coronavirus indicating person-to-person transmission: A study of a family cluster. *Lancet.* 2020;395(10223): 514–523.
3. Chinese Society of Radiology. Radiological diagnosis of COVID-19: First edition of expert recommendations from Chinese Society of Radiology. [Chinese] *Chin J Radiol.* 2020;54: E001.
4. Chung M, Bernheim A, Mei X, *et al.* CT imaging features of 2019 novel coronavirus (2019-nCOV). *Radiol.* February 2020. http://doi.org/10.1148/radiol.2020200230.
5. Guan WJ, Ni ZY, Hu Y, *et al.* Clinical characteristics of coronavirus disease 2019 in China. *N Engl J Med.* February 2020. http://www.nejm.org/doi/full/10.1056/NEJMoa2002032.
6. Henan Medical Association Laboratory Medicine Branch & Henan Provincial Health Commission Clinical Laboratory Centre. Henan Provincial Medical Association Laboratory Medicine Branch and Henan Provincial Health Committee Clinical Laboratory Centre issued the novel coronavirus nucleic acid test specimen detection and biosafety procedures. [Chinese] February 2020. http://www.henanyixue.com/web/01/doc?docId=15809560725 17&itemId=10002.
7. Huang CL, Wang YM, Li XW, *et al.* Clinical features of patients infected with 2019 novel coronavirus in Wuhan, China. *Lancet.* 2020;395(10223): 497–506.

8. Ji JS. *Early CT Signs and Differential Diagnosis of the Novel Coronavirus.* [Chinese] Beijing: Science Press, 2020

9. Li XH, Zeng XS, Liu B, *et al.* COVID-19 infection presenting with CT halo sign. *Radiol.* February 2020. http://pubs.rsna.org/doi/10.1148/ryct.2020200026.

10. Luo WR, Yu H, Gou JZ, *et al.* Clinical pathology of critical patient with novel coronavirus pneumonia (COVID-19). *Preprints 2020,* 2020020407.

11. Ng, MY, Lee, EYP, Yang, J, *et al.* Imaging profile of the COVID-19 infection: Radiologic findings and literature review. *Radiol.* February 2020. http://pubs.rsna.org/doi/10.1148/ryct.2020200034.

12. Notice of Circulation of Diagnosis and Treatment Protocol for Novel Coronavirus Pneumonia (3rd edition) [Chinese]. National Health Commission of the People's Republic of China. January 2020. http://www.gov.cn/zhengce/zhengceku/2020-01/29/content_5472893.htm.

13. Notice of Circulation of Diagnosis and Treatment Protocol for Novel Coronavirus Pneumonia (2nd edition). [Chinese] National Health Commission of the People's Republic of China, January 2020. http://www.nhc.gov.cn/qjjys/s7948/202001/0909555408d842a58828611dde2e6a26.shtml.

14. Notice of Circulation of Diagnosis and Treatment Protocol for Novel Coronavirus Pneumonia (trial version V). [Chinese] National Health Commission of the People's Republic of China, February 2020. http://www.nhc.gov.cn/yzygj/s7653p/202002/3b09b894ac9b4204a79db5b8912d4440.shtml.

15. Pan F, Ye T, Sun P, *et al.* Time course of lung changes on chest CT during recovery from 2019 novel coronavirus (COVID-19) pneumonia. *Radiol.* February 2020. http://pubs.rsna.org.doi/10.1148/radiol.2020200370.

16. Wilson MR, Sample HA, Zorn KC, *et al.* Clinical metagenomic sequencing for diagnosis of meningitis and encephalitis. *N Engl J Med.* 2019;380(24):2327–2340.

17. Wu Y, Xie YL, Wang X. Longitudinal CT findings in COVID-19 pneumonia: case presenting organizing pneumonia pattern. *Radiol.* February 2020. http://pubs.rsna.org/doi/10.1148/ryct.2020200031.

18. Xu Z, Shi L, Wang YJ, *et al.* Pathological findings of COVID-19 associated with acute respiratory distress syndrome. *Lancet Respir Med.* February 2020. http://linkinghub.elsevier.com/retrieve/pii/S2213260020300076X.

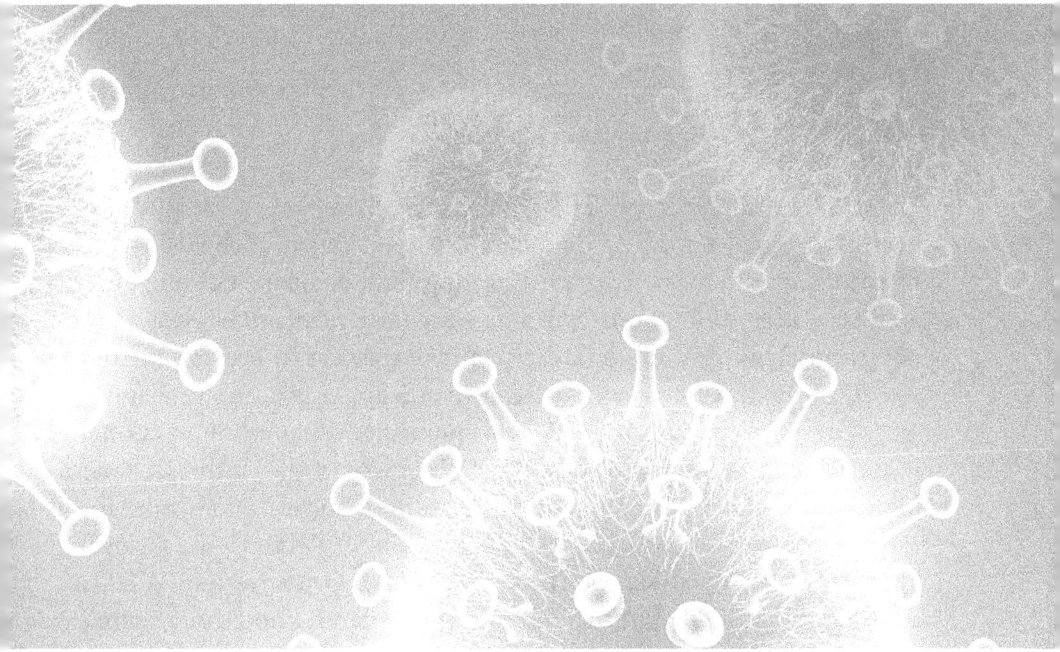

Part 5

Diagnosis and Differential Diagnosis

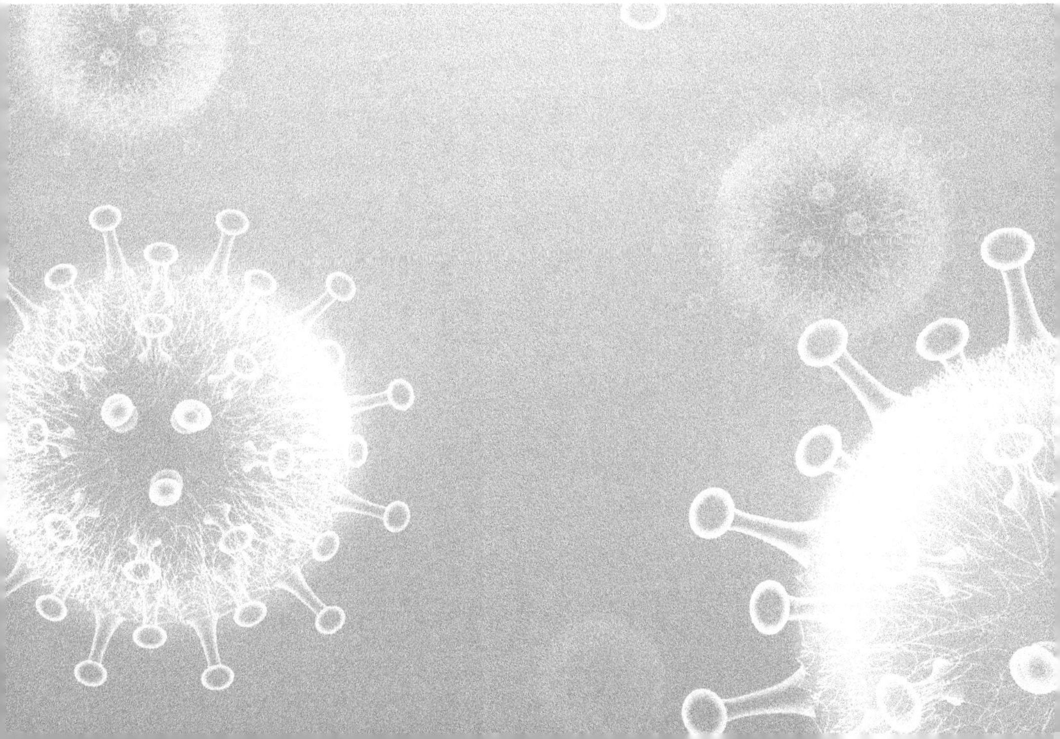

The classic diagnostic model for infectious diseases is to identify suspect cases based on the epidemiological characteristics, clinical manifestations, preliminary laboratory testing, and auxiliary examinations and to screen out confirmed cases accurately through etiological detection. This ideal model can preclude omission to prevent further spread of the disease, as well as achieve efficient and accurate diagnosis. We have fully examined and published the whole genome sequence of SARS-CoV-2 since the early stages of the outbreak, enabling the rapid development and application of nucleic acid testing for early detection of COVID-19 patients. As COVID-19 is a novel infectious disease, China and the World Health Organization (WHO) are improving the diagnostic criteria with in-depth knowledge shared by scientists and clinicians.

Chapter 13
Formulation and Evolution of China's Diagnostic Criteria

After etiological isolation and whole genome sequencing were conducted, the National Health Commission of the People's Republic of China released the first version of *Diagnosis and Treatment Protocol for Novel Coronavirus Pneumonia* on January 15, 2020. It has been further revised five times on January 18, January 22, January 27, February 4, and February 18 (Table 13-1). These publications cover information from the history of contact with the Wuhan seafood market to the confirmation of human-to-human transmission, and record the disease outbreak in Wuhan and its spread to other cities and provinces. The revised diagnostic criteria updated the epidemiological characteristics and the clinical manifestations, which embodied the reflection of epidemiology experts and clinicians on the disease and its countermeasures. These revisions reflect the progress and the accumulation of Chinese experience in the fight against COVID-19.

Table 13-1.   A comparison of 1st–6th versions of diagnostic criteria for COVID-19 released by National Health Commission of the People's Republic of China

Version	Epidemiological History	Clinical Manifestations	Suspected Cases	Confirmed Cases	Clinical Classifications and Definitions
1st	History of travel to Wuhan, or direct/indirect contact with certain markets in Wuhan, especially markets of agricultural products, within two weeks prior to the onset of the disease	1. Fever 2. Radiological characteristics of NCP 3. Normal or decreased leukocyte count, or decreased lymphocyte count in the early stage 4. No obvious improvement or progressive aggravation after three days of standard antibacterial treatment (with reference to *Guidelines for diagnosis and treatment for adult community-acquired pneumonia in China (2016 edition)* released by the Chinese Thoracic Society and *Guidelines for the diagnosis and treatment for children's community-acquired pneumonia (2019 edition)* by the National Health Commission of the People's Republic of China)	Called "observed cases": Consistent with the conditions both of the epidemiological histories and the clinical manifestations	(On the basis of observed cases) Viral gene sequence highly homologous to known novel coronaviruses in the respiratory tract specimens, such as sputum and throat swab according to whole genome sequencing	Definition of critical cases (consistent with any one of the following conditions): 1. Respiratory failure 2. Septic shock 3. Comorbidity with other organ failure and requires ICU monitoring and treatment

| 2nd | 1. History of travel to or residence in Wuhan within 14 days prior to the onset of the disease
Or
2. Contact with patients who have fever and respiratory symptoms from Wuhan within 14 days prior to the onset of the disease
Or
3. Clustered cases | The fourth clinical manifestation in 1st version was removed. | Consistent with the conditions of both the epidemiological histories and the clinical manifestations | RT-PCR showing positive for the novel coronavirus nucleic acid in specimens of suspected cases, such as sputum, throat swab, and lower respiratory secretions; or viral gene sequence highly homologous to known novel coronaviruses according to genome sequencing | Definition of serious cases (consistent with any one of the following conditions):
1. Shortness of breath (breathing rate ≥ 30 times per minute), dyspnea, cyanosis in the lips and mouth; or finger blood oxygen saturation level $\leq 95\%$ during the inhalation of air, or arterial partial pressure of oxygen (PaO_2)/fraction of inspired oxygen $(FiO_2) \leq 300$ mmHg
2. Pulmonary radiology showing multilobar lesions or lesion progression > 50% in 48 hours
3. Quick SOFA (quick Sequential Organ Failure Assessment) score $\geq$ 2 points
4. CURB-65 score ≥ 1 point
5. Comorbid pneumothorax
6. Other clinical conditions requiring hospitalization |
| 3rd | Same as 2nd version | Same as 2nd version | Same as 2nd version | Same as 2nd version | Revised definition of serious cases:
1. Shortness of breath (breathing rate ≥ 30 times per minute), dyspnea, cyanosis in the lips and mouth
2. Finger blood oxygen saturation level $\leq 93\%$ during the inhalation of air
3. Arterial partial pressure of oxygen (PaO_2)/fraction of inspired oxygen $(FiO_2) \leq 300$ mmHg
4. Pulmonary radiology showing multilobar lesions or lesion progression > 50% in 48 hours
5. Other clinical conditions requiring hospitalization |

(Continued)

Table 13-1. (*Continued*)

Version	Epidemiological History	Clinical Manifestations	Suspected Cases	Confirmed Cases	Clinical Classifications and Definitions
4th	Expanding the criteria about contact history to areas outside Wuhan 1. History of travel to or residence in Wuhan or other areas where local cases continue to circulate within 14 days prior to the onset of the disease Or 2. Contact with patients who have fever and respiratory symptoms from Wuhan or other areas where local cases continue to circulate within 14 days prior to the onset of the disease Or 3. Clustered cases or epidemiological association with COVID-19 patients	Same as 2nd version	Loosened criteria for clinical manifestations: consistent with any two conditions of the clinical manifestations and any one of the epidemiological histories	Blood specimens are used for the diagnosis of confirmed cases	Definition of ordinary cases: fever, respiratory symptoms, and radiological characteristics of pneumonia Definition of serious cases was simplified and adjusted slightly, deleting the fourth and the fifth standard in the third version

| 5th (for areas outside Hubei) | 1. History of travel to or residence in Wuhan and its surrounding areas, or in other communities where cases have been reported within 14 days prior to the onset of the disease
Or
2. Contact with lab-confirmed infected patients (with positive results from a nucleic acid test) within 14 days prior to the onset of the disease
Or
3. Contact with patients who have fever or respiratory symptoms from Wuhan and its surrounding areas, or from communities where confirmed cases have been reported within 14 days prior to the onset of disease
Or
4. Clustered cases | Same as 2nd version | Consistent with any one condition of the epidemio-logical histories and any two conditions of the clinical manifestations; or consistent with three conditions of the clinical manifestations and no clear history of epidemiology | Same as 4th version | Definition of ordinary cases: fever, respiratory symptoms, and radiological characteristics of pneumonia
Definition of serious cases was simplified and adjusted slightly, deleting the fourth and the fifth standard in the third version |

Table 13-1. (*Continued*)

Version	Epidemiological History	Clinical Manifestations	Suspected Cases	Confirmed Cases	Clinical Classifications and Definitions
5th (for Hubei)		The criteria for suspected cases were further loosened; Consistent with the conditions of "fever or respiratory symptoms" and "normal or decreased leukocyte count, or decreased lymphocyte count in the early stage"	Consistent with any one condition of the epidemio-logical histories or with no clear history of epidemiology, with two conditions of the clinical manifestations	The introduction of clinical diagnosed cases: suspected cases with the radiological characteristics of NCP	Definition of ordinary cases: fever, respiratory symptoms, and radiological characteristics of pneumonia Definition of serious cases was simplified and adjusted slightly, deleting the fourth and the fifth standard in the third version
6th	Same as 5th version	Same as 2nd version	Consistent with any one condition of the epidemiological histories and any two conditions of the clinical manifestations, or consistent with three conditions of the clinical manifestations and no history of epidemiology	The classification of clinical diagnosed cases specific to Hubei was cancelled	Same as 5th version

13.1 The First Version: Released on January 15, 2020

(1) Observed cases

Consistent with both of the following conditions:

(i) Epidemiological history

History of travel to Wuhan, or direct/indirect contact with certain markets in Wuhan, especially the markets of agricultural products within two weeks prior to the onset of the disease.

(ii) Clinical manifestations

- Fever;
- Radiological characteristics of Novel Coronavirus Pneumonia (NCP);
- Normal or decreased leukocyte count, or decreased lymphocyte count in the early stage;
- No obvious improvement or progressive aggravation after three days of standard antibacterial treatment (with reference to *Guidelines for the Diagnosis and Treatment of Adult Community-acquired Pneumonia in China (2016 edition)* released by the Chinese Thoracic Society and *Guidelines for the Diagnosis and Treatment of Children's Community-acquired Pneumonia (2019 edition)* by the National Health Commission of the People's Republic of China).

(2) Confirmed cases

Viral gene sequence highly homologous to known novel coronaviruses in the respiratory tract specimens, such as sputum and throat swab (on the basis of observed cases) according to whole genome sequencing.

(3) Critical cases

Consistent with any one of the following conditions: respiratory failure, septic shock, or comorbidity of other organ failure that requires ICU monitoring and treatment.

13.2 The Second Version: Detailed Diagnostic Criteria

The first stage of transmission of the novel coronavirus was the local outbreak caused by exposure to the Wuhan seafood market. As increasing observed and confirmed cases had been found, the number of cases with no history of exposure to this market kept rising and clustered cases with no exposure history were discovered, suggesting that the local spread had formed community transmission. Interpersonal transmission and clustered transmission were being found in several communities and families in Wuhan. Confirmed cases from Wuhan with no clear history of exposure to the market were also discovered in several countries and regions outside Mainland China.

In this version, the "observed cases" in the original criteria was renamed "suspect cases"; the epidemiological history of suspect cases was adjusted to history of travel to or residence in Wuhan within two weeks prior to the onset of the disease, or contact with patients with fever and respiratory symptoms from Wuhan within 14 days prior to the onset of the disease, or clustered cases. On account of the high infectivity of the disease, the criterion of the acute clinical judgment after a three-day community-acquired pneumonia (CAP) treatment in the clinical manifestations was deleted, which enhanced the sensitivity of early case detection.

Besides this, the second version has detailed the definitions of serious cases and critical cases respectively in order to distinguish between them.

(1) Suspect cases (previously "observed cases")

Consistent with both of the following conditions:

(i) Epidemiological history

- History of travel to or residence in Wuhan within 14 days prior to the onset of the disease;
- Or contact with patients who have fever and respiratory symptoms from Wuhan within 14 days prior to the onset of the disease;
- Or clustered cases.

(ii) Clinical manifestations

- Fever;
- Radiological characteristics of NCP;
- Normal or decreased leukocyte count, or decreased lymphocyte count in the early stage.

(2) Confirmed cases

On the basis of suspect cases, RT-PCR shows positive for the novel coronavirus nucleic acid in specimens, such as sputum, throat swab, and lower respiratory tract secretions; or viral gene sequence highly homologous to known novel coronaviruses according to genome sequencing.

(3) Serious cases

Consistent with any one of the following conditions:

- Shortness of breath (breathing rate $\geq$ 30 times per minute), dyspnea, cyanosis in the lips and mouth; or finger blood oxygen saturation level $\leq$ 95% during the inhalation of air, or arterial partial pressure of oxygen (PaO_2)/fraction of inspired oxygen (FiO_2) $\leq$ 300 mmHg;
- Pulmonary radiology showing lesions in multiple lobes or lesion progression > 50% in 48 hours;
- Quick SOFA (quick Sequential Organ Failure Assessment) score $\geq$ 2 points;
- CURB-65 score $\geq$ 1 point;
- Comorbid pneumothorax;
- Other clinical conditions requiring hospitalization.

(4) Critical cases

Consistent with any one of the following conditions:

- Respiratory failure;
- Septic shock;
- Comorbidity of other organ failure and requires ICU monitoring and treatment.

13.3 The Third Version: Focus on the Definition of Serious Cases

The third version, released on January 22, 2020, had not revised the section on the epidemiological history. Instead, on the basis of the continuous summary of the clinical characteristics of COVID-19, the third version had revised and simplified the definition of serious cases, such as adjusting the blood oxygen saturation criterion from the previous 95% (in 2nd version) to 93%. Specific criteria are listed as follows:

- Shortness of breath (breathing rate ≥ 30 times per minute), dyspnea, cyanosis in the lips and mouth;
- Finger blood oxygen saturation level ≤ 93% during the inhalation of air;
- Arterial partial pressure of oxygen (PaO_2)/fraction of inspired oxygen (FiO_2) ≤ 300 mmHg;
- Pulmonary radiology showing lesions in multiple lobes or lesion progression > 50% in 48 hours;
- Other clinical conditions requiring hospitalization.

13.4 The Fourth Version: Expanded Scope of Contact History Outside Wuhan

The outbreak of COVID-19 coincided with the Chinese Spring Festival, during which the largest human travel took place. The epidemic rapidly spread beyond Hubei province to other parts of China, and grew into a global pandemic. Following more in-depth understanding of the novel coronavirus and treatment experience, the fourth version released on January 27, 2020 revised the section on epidemiology, expanding the criterion on history of contact to areas outside Wuhan. In addition, blood specimens were used for the diagnosis of confirmed cases for the first time. The definition of ordinary cases was added to the criteria, namely cases with fever, respiratory symptoms, and radiological characteristics of pneumonia. The definition of serious cases was also simplified and modified slightly, with the fourth and the fifth criteria in the third version deleted.

(1) Suspect cases

Consistent with any one condition of the epidemiological histories and any two of the clinical manifestations:

(i) Epidemiological history

- History of travel to or residence in Wuhan or other areas where local cases continue to circulate within 14 days prior to the onset of the disease;

- Contact with patients who have fever and respiratory symptoms from Wuhan or other areas where local cases continue to circulate within 14 days prior to the onset of the disease;
- Clustered cases or epidemiological association with COVID-19 patients.

(ii) Clinical manifestations
- Fever;
- Radiological characteristics of NCP;
- Normal or decreased leukocyte count, or decreased lymphocyte count in the early stage.

(2) Confirmed cases

Real-time fluorescent RT-PCR showing positive for the novel coronavirus nucleic acid in respiratory tract specimens or blood specimens of suspect cases; or viral gene sequence highly homologous to known novel coronaviruses in respiratory tract specimens or blood specimens according to genome sequencing.

(3) Serious cases
- Shortness of breath (breathing rate $\geq$ 30 times per minute), dyspnea, cyanosis in the lips and mouth;
- Finger blood oxygen saturation level $\leq$ 93% during the inhalation of air;
- Arterial partial pressure of oxygen (PaO_2)/fraction of inspired oxygen $(FiO_2) \leq 300$ mmHg.

13.5 The Fifth Version: Clinical Diagnosed Cases in Hubei Province

A large number of cases were discovered in Hubei province, including asymptomatic infected individuals and mild cases, exerting enormous pressure on diagnosis. If patients were not diagnosed, isolated, or treated, second- or third-generation cases would occur. In this sense, clinical manifestations became much more important in the diagnosis of suspect cases. Moreover, the epidemic in Hubei was different from that in other areas of China. Thus, the diagnostic criteria listed differed for cases outside Hubei province and those in Hubei province. For areas outside

Hubei, imported cases still accounted for the largest proportion of the confirmed, while in Hubei, there were a large number of suspect cases to be diagnosed through nucleic acid testing. Furthermore, due to the limited supply and detecting capability of test kits, and the fact that a certain proportion of patients had shown false-negative nucleic acid results, the fifth version introduced "clinically diagnosed" cases in Hubei for the first time. Once a clinically diagnosed case was discovered, medical staff were expected to conduct treatment in isolation immediately and accelerate the collection of specimens for etiological detection in order to minimize possible delays, control the source of infection, and curb the spread of the virus. The introduction of "clinically diagnosed cases" was responsive to the actual situation of the epidemic control and thus improved the diagnosis of the novel coronaviruses. In addition, the criteria for suspect cases were further loosened. The definition of suspect cases only requires "fever or respiratory symptoms" and "normal or decreased leukocyte count, or decreased lymphocyte count in the early stage". The fifth version of the diagnostic criteria are listed as follows:

13.5.1 *Cases outside Hubei province*

(1) Suspect cases

Consistent with any one condition of the epidemiological histories and any two conditions of the clinical manifestations; or consistent with three conditions of the clinical manifestations with no clear history of epidemiology.

(i) Epidemiological history
  - History of travel to or residence in Wuhan and its surrounding areas, or in other communities where cases have been reported within 14 days prior to the onset of the disease;
  - Contact with lab-confirmed infected patients (with positive results from a nucleic acid test) within 14 days prior to the onset of the disease;
  - Contact with patients who have fever or respiratory symptoms from Wuhan and its surrounding areas, or from communities

where confirmed cases have been reported within 14 days prior to the onset of disease;
- Clustered cases.

(ii) Clinical manifestations
- Fever and (or) respiratory symptoms;
- Radiological characteristics of NCP;
- Normal or decreased leukocyte count, or decreased lymphocyte count in the early stage.

13.5.2 *Cases in Hubei province*

(1) Suspect cases

Consistent with any one condition of the epidemiological histories or with no clear history of epidemiology, with two conditions of the clinical manifestations:

(i) Epidemiological history

- History of travel to or residence in Wuhan and its surrounding areas, or in other communities where cases have been reported within 14 days prior to the onset of the disease;
- Contact with lab-confirmed infected patients (with positive results from a nucleic acid test) within 14 days prior to the onset of the disease;
- Contact with patients who have fever or respiratory symptoms from Wuhan and its surrounding areas, or from communities where confirmed cases have been reported within 14 days prior to the onset of disease;
- Clustered cases.

(ii) Clinical manifestations

- Fever and (or) respiratory symptoms;
- Normal or decreased leukocyte count, or decreased lymphocyte count in the early stage.

(2) Clinical diagnosed cases

Suspect cases with radiological characteristics of pneumonia.

Furthermore, the definition of mild cases, namely mild clinical symptoms with no radiological characteristics of pneumonia, was added to the clinical classifications in the fifth version. No modification was made to the definitions of ordinary cases, serious cases, or critical cases.

13.6 The Sixth Version: Clinically Diagnosed Cases Cancelled

Since the release of the fifth version, China had adopted the "four concentration" (concentration of patients, experts, resources, and treatment) principle in comprehensive screening in Hubei province. As a great number of newly established isolation centers and Fangcang shelter hospitals came into use, the detecting capability of nucleic acid testing and the medical supply capacity had been greatly improved. The goal of admitting all patients into medical facilities was gradually achieved and the detecting capability of nucleic acid testing was no longer limiting the diagnosis and treatment of the disease. The classification of clinically diagnosed cases specific to Hubei was cancelled in the sixth version released on February 18, 2020 and the distinction in the diagnostic criteria between Hubei and other areas in China was removed.

(1) Suspect cases

A comprehensive analysis based on the epidemiological histories and the clinical manifestations is required — consistent with any one condition of the epidemiological histories with any two conditions of the clinical manifestations, or consistent with three conditions of the clinical manifestations and no clear history of epidemiology.

(i) Epidemiological history

- History of travel to or residence in Wuhan and its surrounding areas, or in other communities where cases have been reported within 14 days prior to the onset of the disease;
- Contact with lab-confirmed infected patients (with positive results from a nucleic acid test) within 14 days prior to the onset of the disease;

- Contact with patients who have fever or respiratory symptoms from Wuhan and its surrounding areas, or from communities where confirmed cases have been reported within 14 days prior to the onset of disease;
- Clustered cases.

(ii) Clinical manifestations

- Fever and (or) respiratory symptoms;
- Radiological characteristics of NCP;
- Normal or decreased leukocyte count, or decreased lymphocyte count in the early stage.

(2) Confirmed cases

Suspect cases consistent with any one condition of the following etiological evidence:

- RT-PCR showing positive for the novel coronavirus nucleic acid;
- Viral gene sequence highly homologous to known novel coronaviruses according to genome sequencing.

Chapter 14
Draft and Revision of WHO Interim Clinical Care Guidance

On January 12, 2020, the World Health Organization (WHO) released the first draft of *Clinical Management of Severe Acute Respiratory Infection When Novel Coronavirus (nCoV) is Suspected* and revised it on January 28, 2020.

14.1 Definitions for nCoV (Jan 12, 2020)

Suspect case: Severe acute respiratory infection (SARI) in a person, with history of fever and cough requiring admission to hospital, with no other etiology that fully explains the clinical presentation (clinicians should also be alert to the possibility of atypical presentations in patients who are immunocompromised);

AND any of the following:

(1) A history of travel to Wuhan, Hubei province, China, in the 14 days prior to symptom onset;
(2) The disease occurs in a healthcare worker who has been working in an environment where patients with severe acute respiratory infections are being cared for, without regard to place of residence or history of travel;
(3) The person develops an unusual or unexpected clinical course, especially sudden deterioration despite appropriate treatment,

without regard to place of residence or history of travel, even if another etiology has been identified that fully explains the clinical presentation.

A patient with acute respiratory illness of any degree of severity who, within 14 days before the onset of illness, had any of the following exposures:

(1) Close physical contact with a confirmed case of nCoV infection, while that patient was symptomatic;
(2) A healthcare facility in a country where hospital-associated nCoV infections have been reported.

14.2 Definitions for 2019-nCoV (Jan 28, 2020)

14.2.1 *Suspect case*

(1) Patients with severe acute respiratory infection (fever, cough, and requiring admission to hospital) AND with no other etiology that fully explains the clinical presentation AND at least one of the following:

　(i) A history of travel to or residence in the city of Wuhan, Hubei province, China, in the 14 days prior to symptom onset;
　(ii) Patient is a healthcare worker who has been working in an environment where severe acute respiratory infections of unknown etiology are being cared for.

(2) Patients with any acute respiratory illness AND at least one of the followings:

　(i) Close contact with a confirmed or probable case of 2019-nCoV in the 14 days prior to illness onset;
　(ii) Visiting or working in a live animal market in Wuhan, Hubei province, China, in the 14 days prior to symptom onset;
　(iii) Worked or attended a healthcare facility in the 14 days prior to onset of symptoms where patients with hospital-associated 2019-nCoV infections have been reported.

Table 14-1. COVID-19 severity criteria

Infection Type	Criteria
Mild illness	Patients with uncomplicated upper respiratory tract viral infection may have non-specific symptoms such as fever, cough, sore throat, nasal congestion, fatigue, headache, muscle pain, or malaise. The elderly and immunosuppressed may present with atypical symptoms. These patients do not have any signs of dehydration, sepsis, or shortness of breath.
Pneumonia	Patient with pneumonia and no signs of severe pneumonia. Child with non-severe pneumonia has cough or difficulty breathing + fast breathing; fast breathing (in breaths/min): $\geq$ 60 (< 2 months), $\geq$ 50 (2–11 months), $\geq$40 (1–5 years), and no signs of severe pneumonia.
Severe pneumonia	Adolescent or adult: fever or suspected respiratory infection, respiratory rate > 30 breaths/min, severe respiratory distress, or SpO_2 < 90% on room air. Child with cough or difficulty in breathing, plus at least one of the following: central cyanosis or SpO_2 < 90%; severe respiratory distress (e.g., grunting, very severe chest indrawing); signs of pneumonia with a general danger sign: inability to breastfeed or drink, lethargy or unconsciousness, or convulsions. Other signs of pneumonia may be present: chest indrawing, fast breathing (in breaths/min): $\geq$ 60 (< 2 months), $\geq$50 (2–11 months), $\geq$ 40 (1–5 years). The diagnosis is clinical, chest imaging can exclude complications.
Acute respiratory distress syndrome	Onset: new or worsening respiratory symptoms within one week of known clinical insult. Chest imaging (radiograph, CT scan, or lung ultrasound): bilateral opacities, not fully explained by effusions, lobar or lung collapse, or nodules. Origin of edema: respiratory failure not fully explained by cardiac failure or fluid overload. Need objective assessment (e.g., echocardiography) to exclude hydrostatic cause of edema if no risk factor present. Oxygenation (adults): Mild ARDS: 200 mmHg < PaO_2/FiO_2 $\leq$ 300 mmHg (with PEEP or CPAP $\geq$ 5 cmH_2O, or non-ventilated) Moderate ARDS: 100 mmHg < PaO_2/FiO_2 $\leq$ 200 mmHg (with PEEP $\geq$ 5 cmH_2O, or non-ventilated) Severe ARDS: PaO_2/FiO_2 $\leq$ 100 mmHg (with PEEP $\geq$ 5 cmH_2O, or non-ventilated)

(Continued)

Table 14-1. (*Continued*)

Infection Type	Criteria
	When PaO_2 is not available, $SpO_2/FiO_2 \leq 315$ suggests ARDS (including in non-ventilated patients). Oxygenation (children, note OI = Oxygenation Index, and OSI = Oxygenation Index using SpO_2): Bilevel NIV or CPAP ≥ 5 cmH_2O via full face mask: $PaO_2/FiO_2 \leq 300$ mmHg or $SpO_2/FiO_2 \leq 264$ Mild ARDS (invasively ventilated): $4 \leq OI < 8$ or $5 \leq OSI < 7.5$ Moderate ARDS (invasively ventilated): $8 \leq OI < 16$ or $7.5 \leq OSI < 12.3$ Severe ARDS (invasively ventilated): $OI \geq 16$ or $OSI \geq 12.3$.
Sepsis	Adults: life-threatening organ dysfunction. Signs of organ dysfunction include: altered mental status, difficult or fast breathing, low oxygen saturation, reduced urine output, fast heart rate, weak pulse, cold extremities or low blood pressure, skin mottling, or laboratory evidence of coagulopathy, thrombocytopenia, acidosis, high lactate, or hyperbilirubinemia. Children: suspected or proven infection and ≥ 2 SIRS criteria, of which one must be abnormal temperature or white blood cell count.
Septic shock	Adults: persisting hypotension despite volume resuscitation, requiring vasopressors to maintain MAP ≥ 65 mmHg and serum lactate level > 2 mmol/L. Children: any hypotension (SBP < 5th centile or > 2 SD below normal for age) or 2–3 of the following: altered mental state; tachycardia or bradycardia (HR < 90 bpm or > 160 bpm in infants, and HR < 70 bpm or > 150 bpm in children); prolonged capillary refill (> 2 sec) or warm vasodilation with feeble pulses; tachypnea; mottled skin or petechial or purpuric rash; increased lactate; oliguria; hyperthermia or hypothermia.

14.2.2 *Confirmed case*

Collect upper respiratory specimens (nasopharyngeal and oropharyngeal swabs) and lower respiratory specimens (sputum, endotracheal aspirate, or bronchoalveolar lavage) and use RT-PCR to detect 2019-nCoV. If lower respiratory specimens are more accessible (e.g., for ventilated patients, clinicians can choose to collect lower respiratory specimens only). Serological test is only recommended when RT-PCR is unavailable. Table 14-1 presents the severity criteria.

Chapter 15
Differential Diagnosis

SARS-CoV-2 should be differentiated from many other known types of viral pneumonia, including influenza, parainfluenza, adenovirus, respiratory syncytial virus (RSV), rhinovirus, human metapneumovirus, SARS-CoV, mycoplasma pneumonia, chlamydial pneumonia, and bacterial pneumonia. It should also be differentiated from noninfectious diseases such as vasculitis, dermatomyositis, and organizing pneumonia. For clinically diagnosed cases, rapid antigen test and NAAT including multiplexed PCR should be conducted if possible to detect common respiratory pathogens. Coinfection and secondary infection (including nosocomial infection) are possible. Be vigilant about other types of pneumonia during the pandemic.

15.1 Influenza

Influenza is an acute respiratory infectious disease caused by an influenza virus and spread through droplets. Symptoms include acute chills, fever, headache, fatigue, myalgia, and respiratory symptoms. It is highly infectious but self-limiting with a short course. Blood routine index presents decreased total white blood cells and relatively increased lymphocytes. Antigen test or polymerase chain reaction (PCR) test that detects the virus RNA could be used to diagnose the influenza.

15.2 Human Parainfluenza

Human parainfluenza viruses remain the main cause of upper respiratory tract infection and severe lower respiratory tract infection in infants and children. The virus also affects adults and may cause repeated infection. RT-PCR test of virus nucleic acid in nasopharyngeal swabs, oropharyngeal swabs, and bronchoalveolar lavage fluids is currently the main rapid test method.

15.3 Adenovirus Infection

Adenoviruses are spread primarily in winter and spring. Humans of all ages could be infected, but infants, the elderly, and immunocompromised individuals are more easily infected. The virus causes a wide range of illnesses, from acute upper respiratory tract infection to pneumonia, and is highly infective. The virus can be identified with qPCR.

15.4 RSV Infection

Human respiratory syncytial virus is a major cause of acute respiratory tract infection in infants, commonly seen in autumn and winter. Infected children and adults may present mild upper respiratory tract symptoms, while infected elderly may present pneumonia or other severe illnesses. RT-PCR is currently the most common test method.

15.5 Rhinovirus Infection

The rhinovirus is the predominant cause of the common cold usually seen in spring and autumn, and often causes repeated infection. Symptoms include nasal congestion, sore throat, sneezing, and hoarseness, sometimes accompanied by mild body symptoms without apparent infection symptoms.

15.6 Human Metapneumovirus Infection

Symptoms of human metapneumovirus infection range from upper respiratory tract infection to severe bronchiolitis and pneumonia.

Infection tends to occur frequently in winter and spring (with differences between northern and southern hemispheres). Children and the elderly are more easily infected. RT-PCR is currently the key test method.

15.7 SARS

SARS has similar early symptoms with SARS-CoV-2, including fever, arthralgia, myalgia, and lethargy. Patients may cough but then rapidly develop pulmonary inflammatory changes that lead to chest distress and shortness of breath. Peripheral blood lymphocytes decrease. It can be identified with serology and viral nucleic acid test.

15.8 Mycoplasma Pneumonia

Mycoplasma pneumoniae is an important pathogen that causes 5–30% of community-acquired pneumonia (CAP), with children and adolescents the most susceptible. Symptoms are relatively mild, mainly dry cough. Chest signs are few, but imaging diagnosis shows severe and diverse changes, and ground-glass opacities. Peripheral leukocytosis is not clear. Serological test of the IgM antibody in the acute stage remains the most important diagnostic approach, while nucleic acid test could be used in early rapid diagnosis.

15.9 Chlamydia Pneumonia

Chlamydia pneumoniae is an important pathogen that causes CAP and about 10% of pneumonia cases that are transferred to another hospital. Symptoms are non-specific, ranging from mild to severe, while infected seniors often develop severe symptoms. Early stage presentations are upper respiratory tract infection, commonly with a sore throat; late stage presentations include fever and cough (mainly dry cough). Laboratory examinations often return normal results, with imaging examinations showing non-specific features. Serological test is the most common, specific, and sensitive method, while nucleic acid test could be used as an early stage rapid diagnosis method.

15.10 Bacterial Pneumonia

Bacterial pneumonia often develops into fever, cough, and expectoration. Cough starts from dry cough, and develops into expectoration, with sputum often purulent or ferruginous. Laboratory test discovers increased leukocyte count and neutrophil elevation. Antibiotic therapy is normally effective.

15.11 Vasculitis

A patient with the antineutrophil cytoplasmic antibody (ANCA)-related vasculitis may present respiratory tract symptoms, including running nose, nasosinusitis, cough, hemoptysis, chest distress, shortness of breath, and pulmonary shadow, sometimes involving multiple systemic organs. Laboratory tests often present leukocytosis, elevated eosinophils, and ANCA positive. Imaging test is of importance. Tissue biopsy could aid in diagnosis.

15.12 Dermatomyositis

A patient with dermatomyositis and pulmonary symptoms may have interstitial pneumonia, particularly for patients with positive Anti Jo-1 antibody. CT lung scanning presents ground-glass opacities, lineal shadows, and patchy consolidation. Patients may develop difficult breathing and hypoxemia. A patient with dermatomyositis and interstitial pneumonia often present skin lesion and myositis. Laboratory test may discover positive myositis-related antibodies and elevated level of serum muscle enzymes.

15.13 Cryptogenic Organizing Pneumonia

Patients with cryptogenic organizing pneumonia (COP) present diverse symptoms, mostly subacute process and influenza-like symptoms, including fever, cough, and mild to medium shortness of breath. A small number may experience severe breathing difficulty.

Most patients present general malaise, appetite loss, and weight loss. Two thirds of the patients have Velcro rale in lung auscultation. Imaging findings have non-specific certain features. Pathological diagnosis can be helpful. Causes for COP should be proactively investigated. Hormone therapy is effective.

References

1. Chen, H. *Practical Internal Medicine*. [Chinese] Beijing: People's Medical Publishing House. 2017.
2. Notice of Circulation of Diagnosis and Treatment Protocol for Novel Coronavirus Pneumonia (Trial 6th Edition). [Chinese] National Health Commission of the People's Republic of China, Office of the National Administration of Traditional Chinese Medicine, February 2020. http://www.nhc.gov.cn/yzygj/s7653p/202002/8334a8326dd94d329df351d7da8aefc2.shtml.
3. Notice of Circulation of Diagnosis and Treatment Protocol for Novel Coronavirus Pneumonia (Trial 3rd Edition). [Chinese] National Health Commission of the People's Republic of China, January 2020. http://www.nhc.gov.cn/yzygj/s7653p/202001/f492c9153ea9437bb587ce2f-fcbee1fa.shtml.
4. Notice of Circulation of Diagnosis and Treatment Protocol for Novel Coronavirus Pneumonia (Trial 4th Edition). [Chinese] National Health Commission of the People's Republic of China, January 2020. http://www.nhc.gov.cn/yzygj/s7653p/202001/4294563ed35b43209b31739bd0785e67.shtml.
5. Notice of Circulation of Diagnosis and Treatment Protocol for Novel Coronavirus Pneumonia (Trial 5th Edition). [Chinese] National Health Commission of the People's Republic of China, February 2020. http://www.nhc.gov.cn/yzygj/s7653p/202002/3b09b894ac9b4204a79db5b8912d44.shtml.
6. Diagnosis and Treatment Protocol for Novel Coronavirus Pneumonia (Trial). [Chinese] National Health Commission of the People's Republic of China, January 2020.
7. Diagnosis and Treatment Protocol for Novel Coronavirus Pneumonia (Trial 2nd Edition). [Chinese] National Health Commission of the People's Republic of China, January 2020.

8. Clinical management of severe acute respiratory infection when novel coronavirus (nCoV) infection is suspected: Interim Guidance. [Chinese] World Health Organization, January 2020. http://www.who.int/publications-detail/clinical-management-of-severe-acute-respiratory-infection-when-novel-coronavirus-(ncov)-infection-is-suspected.

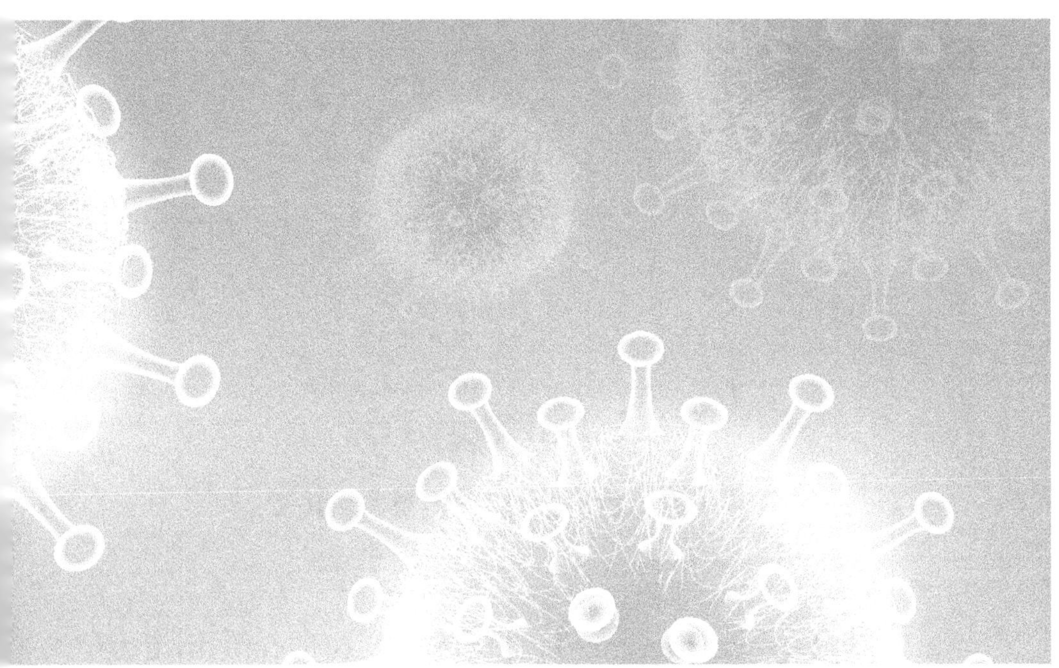

Part 6

Treatment Principles and Progress in Drug Research

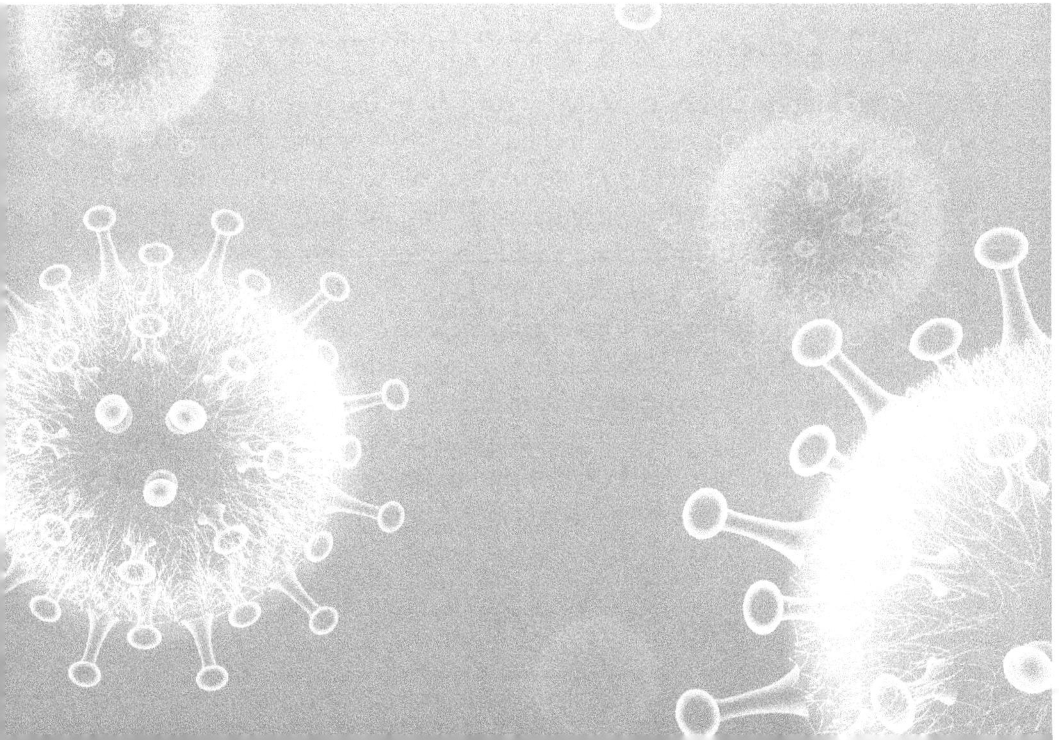

Chapter 16
Treatment Principles

16.1 Determine the Treatment Site According to Patients' Conditions

Suspected and confirmed COVID-19 patients should be quarantined and treated in designated hospitals with effective quarantine and protection conditions. Each suspected patient should be isolated and treated in a single room, while more than one confirmed patient can be admitted to the same ward. Patients in critical conditions should be admitted to ICU as early as possible.

16.2 General Treatment Principles

Treatment should be provided according to the severity of the conditions. Patients should rest in bed, receive supportive treatment and adequate calories; fluid and electrolyte balance should be maintained to keep the internal environment stable; and vital signs and finger pulse oxygen saturation rate should be closely monitored. Complete blood count (CBC), clinical urine tests, C-reactive protein (CRP), biochemical indicators (liver enzyme, myocardial enzyme, kidney function, etc.), coagulation function, and other indicators should be examined. Chest imaging and arterial blood gas analysis should be conducted. Effective oxygen therapy, including nasal catheter, mask oxygen inhalation, and high-flow nasal cannula oxygen therapy (HFNC) should be administered in a timely manner.

16.3 Discharge Criteria

Those who meet all the following conditions can be considered for discharge: body temperature has returned to normal for more than three days; respiratory symptoms significantly improved; tangible improvement in acute exudative lesions in pulmonary imaging; negative result in nucleic acid test of respiratory tract specimen for two consecutive times (sampling time shall be at least one day apart); and the total course of the disease was more than two weeks.

16.4 Health Management of Discharged Patients

Patients discharged from the hospital should still be closely followed up. Follow-up visits to designated outpatient clinics are recommended in the second and the fourth week after discharge. When a patient is discharged from the hospital, his or her residential address should be confirmed. After discharge, the patient should rest at home for two weeks and avoid activities in public places. It is necessary to wear a mask when going out.

Chapter 17
Progress in Research of Antiviral Drugs

As of February 2020, there has been no proven effective anti-virus therapy. Since the outbreak of COVID-19 in January 2020, researchers and clinicians all over the world have been focusing on the research and development of antiviral drugs. A large number of conventional drugs in new use and new drugs in clinical trial stage II and III have been registered for clinical research for controlled study in the treatment of COVID-19. However, according to the experience of SARS and MERS as well as the normal cycle of clinical drug development, it is hard to develop drugs that are definitely effective, safe, and capable of being mass-produced for clinical treatment within a short time. This chapter introduces the ideas of screening anti-coronavirus drugs, potential drugs selected from *in vitro* tests, and the general situation of drugs that are currently under clinical research.

17.1 Methods for Screening Anti-coronavirus Drugs

Prior to 2003, there were only two pathogenic coronaviruses, CoV-229E and CoV-OC43, which usually caused self-limited upper respiratory tract infections. Therefore, the sudden outbreak of SARS-CoV in 2003 caught researchers and institutions, especially those involved in antiviral development, ill-prepared. Since then, researchers around the world have used three common approaches to find potential antiviral drugs against coronaviruses.

The first approach is to test broad-spectrum antiviral drugs used to treat other viral infections by conducting standard assays that measure the effects of these drugs on the cytotoxicity, production of virus, and formation of plaque in living viruses or pseudocoronaviruses (which have a portion of the coronavirus structure) in living cells. Examples of drugs identified with this method include interferon (IFN-α, IFN-β, IFN-γ), ribavirin, and cyclophilin inhibitors. These drugs are readily available with known pharmacokinetic and pharmacodynamic properties, adverse reactions, and dosage regimens, which make them distinctly advantageous. However, they generally have no specific anti-coronavirus effect and may be associated with severe adverse reactions.

The second approach to find anti-coronavirus drugs involves screening compound libraries that encompass abundant existing compounds and databases, which contain information about transcriptional characteristics in different cell lines. This method allows for rapid, high-throughput screening of many readily available compounds, which can then be further evaluated with antiviral assays. Various drugs have been identified in these drug reuse programs, including many with crucial physiological and/or immunological effects, such as affecting neurotransmitter regulation, estrogen receptors, kinase signaling, lipid or sterol metabolism, protein processing and DNA synthesis or repair. The main drawback of the approach, however, is that although many identified drugs have shown anti-coronavirus activity *in vitro*, for most drugs, the half maximal effective concentration (EC50) related to immune inhibition or anti-coronavirus is significantly higher than the maximum serum concentrations (C_{max}) in therapeutic doses. As a result, these drugs have no actual clinical application value. The anti-HIV protease inhibitor lopinavir/ritonavir, however, is one of the few exceptions that has been tested effective in both non-human primate models and non-randomized clinical trials.

The third approach involves newly developed specific drugs based on the understanding of genomes and the molecular structure of individual coronavirus. These drugs include siRNA molecules or inhibitors targeting specific viral enzymes involved in viral replication cycle, mAb targeting host receptors, protease inhibitors of host cells, inhibitors of virus endocytosis by host cells, human or humanized mAb targeting S1 subunit (receptor-binding domain), and antiviral peptide targeting S2 subunit. Despite the fact that most of these drugs have effective anti-coronavirus activity *in vitro* and/or *in vivo*, their pharmacokinetic and pharmacodynamic properties and adverse reactions are yet to be evaluated in animal and human trials. In addition, it often takes years to develop these drug candidates into clinically useful treatment options with a reliable mode of administration to patients.

The three approaches generally go hand in hand during outbreaks of novel coronavirus for the selection of candidate pharmaceutical compounds that can be broadly divided into virus-based and host-based as treatment options.

17.2 Potential Drugs for the Treatment of SARS-CoV-2

17.2.1 *Drugs targeting the virus*

The approved nucleoside analogues favipiravir and ribavirin, and the ones under tests, remdisivir and galidesivir, may have the potential to resist SARS-CoV-2. RNA-dependent RNA polymerase (RdRp) is an important component of the coronavirus replication and transcription complex, and participates in the production of genomic and subgenomic RNA. Nucleoside analogues in the form of adenine or guanine derivatives target RdRp and block the synthesis of viral RNA in various RNA viruses, including human coronavirus.

17.2.1.1 *Ribavirin*

Ribavirin is a guanine analogue with broad-spectrum antiviral activity that has been applied in the treatment of severe RSV infection, viral hepatitis C, and viral hemorrhagic fever. Its exact mechanism of action remains unclear, but for RNA viruses (including coronaviruses), the inhibition of mRNA upper limit and the induction of mutations in RNA-dependent viral replication are considered important. High doses of ribavirin have been used to treat SARS patients, but the efficacy is yet to be studied. It showed moderate anti-MERS-CoV activity at high doses and in rhesus monkeys infected with MERS-CoV, but no significant survival benefit was observed in small groups of MERS patients. Moreover, serious adverse reactions associated with large doses of ribavirin limits its clinical application in serious patients with COVID-19.

17.2.1.2 *Favipiravir (T-705)*

Favipiravir is a guanine analogue approved for the treatment of influenza that effectively inhibits the RdRp of various RNA viruses such as influenza, Ebola, yellow fever, chikungunya, norovirus, and enterovirus. A recent study reported that it can inhibit the *in vitro* activity of SARS-CoV-2 (EC_{50} = 61.88 μM in Vero E6 cells). A number of clinical randomized controlled trials of COVID-19 are being conducted to evaluate the efficacy of the combination of favipiravir with IFN-α and of favipiravir with baloxavir marbolix (an approved influenza inhibitor for cap-snatching).

17.2.1.3 *Remdesivir (GS-5734)*

Remdesivir is a phosphoramidate prodrug of adenine derivative. Its chemical structure is similar to that of tenofovir alafenamide, an approved HIV reverse transcriptase inhibitor. Remdesivir has demonstrated broad-spectrum activity against RNA viruses such as SARS-CoV and MERS-CoV in cell cultures and animal models. In clinical trials of Ebola, however, the results have been poor. A recent study showed that remdesivir could inhibit SARS-CoV-2 (EC_{50} = 0.77 μm in Vero E6 cells) *in vitro*. According to a report in the *New England Journal of Medicine*, a COVID-19 patient in the United States recovered after receiving intravenous injection of remdesivir on Feb 4, 2020. Thus, the drug appeared to have improved clinical outcomes.

Two phase III trials have been conducting from early February 2020 to evaluate the efficacy and safety of remdesivir through intravenous injection on COVID-19 patients (200 mg on day 1, 100 mg per day on day 2-9, once per day for nine days). The estimated time of completion is April 2020. One of the trials involving 761 patients was conducted in a randomized, placebo-controlled, double-blind approach in various hospitals in Wuhan, China.

17.2.1.4 *Galidesivir (BCX4430)*

Galidesivir is an adenosine analogue originally developed for hepatitis C virus. It acts as a non-obligate RNA chain terminator to inhibit the RdRp of broad-spectrum RNA viruses, including coronaviruses (such as SARS-CoV and MERS-CoV) and filoviruses (such as Ebola and Marburg virus). The drug has been rapidly moved into clinical trials to expand treatment options for the Ebola virus in Africa.

17.2.1.5 *Lopinavir and Ritonavir*

Researches show that lopinavir-ritonavir, an approved protease inhibitor against HIV, is active against SARS and MERS. Lopinavir-ritonavir exhibited anti-coronavirus activity *in vitro* as well as in SARS patients and in non-randomized trials on non-human primates infected with MERS-CoV. It is speculated that the 3CL inhibitory activity of lopinavir-ritonavir contributes at least in part to its anti-coronavirus effect. Clinical trials have been initiated to test the efficacy and safety of HIV protease inhibitors, such as lopinavir-ritonavir, in patients infected with SARS-CoV-2. The clinical trial hypothesized that lopinavir-ritonavir could inhibit 3C-like proteinase (3CLpro inhibitor) in SARS and MERS, and appeared to be associated with improved clinical outcomes in SARS patients in a non-randomized open study.

However, it remains to be seen whether the routine use of lopinavir-ritonavir in the treatment of coronavirus infections will develop resistance the same way it did in the treatment of HIV-infected patients. In addition, it is still controversial whether HIV protease inhibitors can effectively inhibit the 3CL hydrolase (3CLpro) and papain-like protease (PLpro) of SARS-CoV-2. HIV protease belongs to the aspartic protease family, while two coronavirus proteases come from the cysteine protease family. When developed, this class of drugs was optimized specifically for HIV protease inhibitors to suit the C2 symmetry of the catalytic site of the HIV protease dimer, but there is no such C2 symmetric pocket structure in coronavirus proteases. Their efficacy remains a problem if HIV protease inhibitors alter host pathways to indirectly interfere with coronavirus infection. Recently, a clinical study of the efficacy of lopinavir-ritonavir and arbidol in the treatment of COVID-19 showed that the two drugs were not found to improve symptoms or shorten the time of negative conversion of viral nucleic acid in respiratory specimens.

17.2.1.6 *Griffithsin*

Spike glycoprotein (protein S) is also a potential therapeutic target. Griffithsin is a lectin derived from red algae that binds to oligosaccharides on the surface of various viral glycoproteins, including HIV gp120 and SARS-CoV protein S. In SARS-CoV-infected mice and *in vitro*, griffithsin specifically binds to glycoproteins on the surface of the virus, such as protein S and HIV gp120 protein. It inhibits a wide range of oligosaccharides in coronavirus, including SARS-CoV, CoV-229E, CoV-OC43, and CoV-NL63. Griffithsin has been tested as HIV prevention gel or enema in phase I study. The safety of these drugs and their optimal way of delivery in the body should be further evaluated in the treatment or prevention of SARS-CoV-2.

17.2.1.7 *Monoclonal antibodies*

The combination of neutralizing monoclonal antibodies REGN3048 and REGN3051 is being studied against coronavirus infection in the first human clinical trial funded by the National Institute of Allergy and Infectious Diseases (NIAID). The safety and tolerance of the drug will be studied in 48 patients. Both antibodies bind to the protein S of MERS-CoV. In a mouse model of MERS, intravenous injection of the drug can neutralize MERS-CoV at high levels in circulating blood and reduce viral load in the lungs.

17.2.1.8 *Targeted therapy based on CRISPR/Cas13d technology*

The CRISPR/Cas13d system may be a direct, flexible, and rapid novel approach for the treatment and prevention of RNA virus infection. This system can be used to specifically target the RNA genome of SARS-CoV-2, thereby limiting its replication ability. An advantage of the CRISPR/Cas13d system is its flexibility in RNA-guiding and RNA-targeting, since the RNA-target cleavage activity of CRISPR/Cas13d is independent of the presence of specific adjacent sequences. Due to the pulmonary eosinophilic characteristics of adeno-associated viral vector (AAV), it can be used as a carrier for targeted drug delivery of CRISPR system. Further studies are needed to ensure the safety and efficacy of the system in eliminating SARS-CoV-2 and other viruses in animal models before therapeutic applications can be made in patients.

17.2.2 *Drugs targeting the host*

17.2.2.1 *Interferon (IFN)*

The host's intrinsic IFN response is essential for controlling viral replication after infection. Although coronaviruses can suppress the immune evasive IFN response, they are still susceptible to IFN treatment *in vitro*. The IFN response can be reinforced by the administration of recombinant IFN or an IFN inducer. Recombinant IFN-α and IFN-β inhibit the replication of SARS-CoV and MERS-CoV both *in vitro* and in animal models. The combinations of IFN-α or IFN-β with other antiviral drugs such as ribavirin and/or lopinavir-ritonavir have been used to treat patients with SARS or MERS. Overall, however, the combination treatment of IFN and ribavirin cannot consistently improve prognosis.

Pegylated IFNα-2a (PEG-IFNα-2a) and pegylated IFNα-2b (PEG-IFNα-2b) approved for the treatment of hepatitis B virus (HBV) and hepatitis C virus (HCV) can be used to stimulate the innate antiviral response in patients infected with SARS-CoV-2. Trials involving IFN, including the anti-HCV combination therapy with PEG-IFN and ribavirin, have been initiated. It is not clear whether

PEG-IFN and nucleoside compounds have synergistic effect against SARS-CoV-2. Due to multiple adverse reactions of IFN treatment, it should be closely monitored and evaluated. Furthermore, dose reduction or termination of treatment may be necessary.

17.2.2.2 *Baricitinib*

ACE2 is considered to be the receptor of SARS-CoV-2 infecting pneumocytes. Over 80% of ACE2 in lung is distributed on the surface of ATII cells. Other organs that express ACE2 include the kidney, heart, and blood vessels. These ATII cells are particularly vulnerable to viral infection. One of the known endocytosis regulatory factor is AP2-accociated kinase 1 (AAK1), the destruction of which may, in turn, interrupt the transmission of the virus to cells and the intracellular assembly of virus particles. Among the known AAK1 inhibitors, six have been found to inhibit AAK1 with high affinity. The JAK kinase inhibitor, baricitinib, received much attention because the plasma concentration at therapeutic dose of baricitinib (1 dose per day, 2 mg or 4 mg each time) is sufficient to inhibit AAK1.

So far, these compounds targeting receptors have not been tested in patients infected with coronavirus. Their anti-coronavirus activity may be narrow-spectrum because different coronaviruses use different host cell receptors. In addition, immunopathologic risks must be assessed, particularly in view of the multiple biological and immunological functions of these receptors.

17.2.2.3 *Chloroquine*

Chloroquine is a 4-aminoquinoline drug that has been considered as a classic antimalarial drug since its discovery in 1934. Chloroquine was the first drug to be mass-produced for the prevention and control of malaria infection. Chloroquine is active in fighting red cell stage *Plasmodium ovale, P. malariae,* and the sensitive *P. vivax* and *P. falciparum.* With high volume of distribution, chloroquine can infiltrate into most tissues and the serum drug concentration can be maintained for up to two months. Adverse reactions to chloroquine include headache, dizziness, abdominal discomfort, vomiting, and diarrhea, but serious adverse reactions are extremely rare. Chloroquine is available only through oral medication while significant toxicity can be caused through intravenous infusion.

In recent years, chloroquine has been found to be an inhibitor of endosome acidification, which can isolate protons to lysosomes to increase the pH of cells and thus resisting the infection of certain viruses. It is also suggested that inhibition of glycosylation may be the main mechanism of antiviral action of chloroquine. In addition, chloroquine has immunomodulatory effects, inhibiting the production and release of TNF-α and IL-6, which are involved in mediating the inflammatory response of viral infection. It has broad-spectrum antiviral activity *in vitro* against a variety of coronaviruses (SARS-CoV, MERS-CoV, CoV-229E and CoV-OC43) and other RNA viruses, including flavivirus and HIV. Recent studies have shown an inhibitory effect on SARS-CoV-2 (EC_{50} = 1.13 μM in Vero-E6 cells). However, possibly because the pathway of cell surface was not simultaneously blocked, it did not substantially reduce the virus replication in SARS-CoV infected mice in previous animal experiments. So far, various institutions in China have adopted chloroquine phosphate or hydroxychloroquine as one of the drugs in combination treatment program or intervention to conduct open research to evaluate the efficacy of chloroquine and its structural analogues.

17.2.2.4 *Nitazoxanide*

Approved for the treatment of diarrhea, nitazoxanide can also inhibit SARS-CoV-2 *in vitro* (EC50 = 2.12 μM in Vero E6 cells). The antiviral effect of the drug also needs to be evaluated in clinical studies.

17.3. Limitations of Existing Drugs

Despite a large number of reports on virus-based and host-based treatment regimens, they show strong *in vitro* activity against SARS and MERS. The activity against SARS-CoV-2 has been studied *in vitro* with good results, but only a few regimens can realize its clinical potential in the foreseeable future.

Most drugs have one or more major limitations and cannot be continued *in vitro*. Firstly, many drugs, including cyclosporine, chlorpromazine and IFN-α, have high EC_{50}/C_{max} ratios at clinically relevant doses. Secondly, some drugs can cause serious side effects or immunosuppression. For example, hemolytic anemia, neutropenia, teratogenicity, and cardiopulmonary distress may be associated with the use of large doses of ribavirin. Fatal infection happened in macaques infected with MERS-CoV after they were treated with mycophenolate mofetil (MMF). Viral load in their lungs and extrapulmonary tissue was then even higher than that in the untreated control group. Immunopathology can be induced by drugs that target host signaling pathways or receptors. Moreover, the lack of reliable drug delivery approaches *in vivo* is also a problem for siRNA and other drugs that have not previously been used in humans.

17.4 Conclusion and Outlook

Rapid screening of effective interventions against SARS-CoV-2 is a major challenge. Given the current knowledge of their safety and, in some cases, their efficacy against coronaviruses closely related to SARS-CoV-2, reusing existing antiviral drugs is a potentially important near-term strategy for resisting SARS-CoV-2.

The phase III clinical trial of remdesivir has been started. Clinical trials on umifenovir, oseltamivir and darunavir/cobicistat are also being conducted in China, although there has been no sufficient information to prove their potential antiviral activity against coronavirus. In addition, existing MERS and/or SARS inhibitors can be screened by SARS-CoV-2. But the EC_{50} and IC_{50} values of the inhibitors are usually within the micromole range, with no guarantee of their activity against SARS-CoV-2. As a result, the existing MERS and/or SARS inhibitors can accept clinical evaluation on efficacy and safety in humans only after passing through both cell and animal screenings.

In an epidemic outbreak, "compassionate use" and "off-label use" are allowed under the state of emergency before new drugs come into market, but adherence to the basic principles of clinical research is essential to ensure that investigational drugs are properly evaluated. Clinical trials must be conducted under the principles of randomization, control, and repetition. The evaluation index should be as objective as possible and blinded evaluation should be adopted if possible. In accordance with the statistical guidance of clinical trials, sufficient sample size should be guaranteed, the control group should be set reasonably, the grouping should be truly randomized and deviation should be avoided.

In summary, no antiviral drugs against coronavirus, including SARS-CoV-2, have been confirmed effective as of February 2020. The global outbreak of COVID-19 urgently requires the joint efforts of all countries in the world to develop broad-spectrum antiviral drugs against coronavirus. In the long run, the development of new broad-spectrum antiviral drugs that work against a variety of coronaviruses may be the ultimate treatment strategy for infections caused by sustained transmission and novel coronaviruses.

Chapter 18
Precautions for the Treatment
of Special Population

18.1 Children

Most confirmed pediatric cases exhibit mild clinical symptoms and have a relatively clear epidemiological history. Still, doctors should closely observe the progress of pediatric patients' conditions, regularly monitor their vital signs and peripheral oxygen saturation (SpO_2), etc., and identify the severe and critical cases as early as possible. Doctors should also develop a treatment plan based on the severity of patients' conditions. For instance, for upper respiratory tract infection and mild pneumonia, symptomatic/supportive treatment is advised. Such treatment includes maintaining a regular daily schedule and ensuring sufficient sleep; balancing the diet, enhancing nutritional support, and ensuring sufficient calorie intake; attending to water and electrolyte balance; and offering psychotherapies, etc. None of the reported antiviral medicines thus far has had medical evidence guiding their pediatric use. For patients with mild pathological change on lung tissues and no evidence of bacterial infection, the use of antibacterial agents is not advised. If the pulmonary lesions or pulmonary wet crackles are obvious or there exists evidence of bacterial coinfection, empirical use of antibacterial agents will be suggested. Assessment should be done in the subsequent 48-72 hours; if the possibility of bacterial coinfection is ruled out, antibacterial agents should no longer be applied. The use of glucocorticoids is not normally recommended. The severe and critical cases of pediatric patients should be treated in accordance with relevant routines of diagnosis and treatment.

18.2 Pregnant Women

It is advisable to admit and treat pregnant women infected with COVID-19 in designated hospitals equipped to effectively quarantine and protect patients and medical staff. The pregnant patients should be administered jointly by relevant divisions, including the Division of Infectious Diseases, the Division of Obstetrics & Gynecology, and ICUs, etc. The use of FDA Pregnancy Category D drugs should be avoided as much as possible in the antiviral treatment. If the use of antibacterial agents is necessary, it will be advised to select FDA Category B drugs. If the gestation has continued for less than 28 weeks, anti-infection treatment should be considered as the primary treatment, and the gestation may continue if the patient's condition is under control; if the condition quickly worsens, joint decisions made by the Division of Obstetrics & Gynecology, the Division of Anesthesia, the operating room (OR), the Division of Respiration , the Division of Infectious Diseases, the Division of Neonatology, the Infection-control Department, and the Office of Hospital Administration will be necessary.

18.3 Newborns

All suspected or confirmed cases of newborns should be admitted to neonatal units as early as possible for monitoring and treatment. Clinically, symptomatic/supportive treatment is advised as the primary treatment. The homeostasis of the patients should be maintained, and trachea interventional operations should be avoided as much as possible. Medical institutions should arrange for effective single room accommodation and take contact precautions and droplet precautions. They should take airborne precautions when their operation is likely to produce aerosols. Newborns are advised to be quarantined for 10–14 days. Breastfeeding will not be advised until the mothers' recovery. During the treatment, newborns should be closely monitored, and protective measures of quarantine should be taken in the process of referral. To date, there has not been any effective medicine against coronaviruses. Doctors should also avoid arbitrary or inappropriate use of antibacterial agents on newborns.

References

1. Barnard DL, Day CW, Bailey K, *et al.* Evaluation of immunomodulators, interferons and known *in vitro* SARS-CoV inhibitors for inhibition of SARS-CoV replication in BALB/c mice. *Antivir Chem Chemother.* 2006;17(5):275–84.
2. Brown AJ, Won JJ, Graham RL, *et al.* Broad spectrum antiviral remdesivir inhibits human endemic and zoonotic deltacoronaviruses with a highly divergent RNA dependent RNA polymerase. *Antiviral Research.* 2019;169:104541.
3. Cai J, Xu J, Lin D, *et al.* A case series of children with 2019 novel coronavirus infection: Clinical and epidemiological features. *Clin Infect Dis.* 2020;ciaa198.
4. Chen F, Hao Y, Zhang Z, *et al.* An urgent call for raising the scientific rigorousness of clinical trials on COVID-19. [Chinese]. *Chin J Epidemiol.* 2020;41(3):301–2.
5. Chen J, Ling Y, Xi X, *et al.* Efficacies of lopinavir/ritonavir and abidol in the treatment of novel coronavirus pneumonia. *Chin J Infect Dis.* 2020;38. http://rs.yiigle.com/yufabiao/1182592.htm
6. Children's Hospital of Fudan University, Guideline-making team for the quick screening and management of children with suspected or confirmed COVID-19. Quick screening and management of children with suspected or confirmed COVID-19: A rapid advice guideline. [Chinese]. *Chin. J. Evid. Based Pediatr* 2020;15(1):1–4.
7. del Rio C, Malani PN. 2019 novel coronavirus — important information for clinicians. *JAMA.* 2020;323(11):1039–40.
8. Holshue ML, DeBolt C, Lindquist S, *et al.* First case of 2019 novel coronavirus in the United States. *N Engl J Med.* 2020;382(10):929–36.
9. Keyaerts E, Li S, Vijgen L, *et al.* Antiviral activity of chloroquine against human coronavirus OC43 infection in newborn mice. *Antimicrob. Agents Chemother.* 2009;53(8):3416–21.

10. Li X, Zheng J, Xu Y. Guangdong province expert consensus on the pediatric diagnosis and treatment of 2019-novel coronavirus pneumonia. [Chinese]. *Guangdong Med. J.* 2020;41(3):217–21.

11. Morse JS, Lalonde T, Xu S, Liu WR. Learning from the past: Possible urgent prevention and treatment options for severe acute respiratory infections caused by 2019-nCoV. *Chembiochem.* 2020;21(5):730–8.

12. Nguyen TM, Zhang Y, Pandolfi PP. Virus against virus: A potential treatment for 2019-nCov (SARS-CoV-2) and other RNA viruses. *Cell Res.* 2020;30(3):189–90.

13. Pediatric Branch of Hubei Medical Association, Pediatric Branch of Wuhan Medical Association, Pediatric Medical Quality Control Center of Hubei. Recommendation for the diagnosis and treatment of novel coronavirus infection in children in Hubei (Trial version 1). [Chinese]. *Chin. J. Contemp. Pediatr.* 2020;22(2):96–9.

14. Richardson P, Griffin I, Tucker C, *et al.* Baricitinib as potential treatment for 2019-nCoV acute respiratory disease. *Lancet.* 2020;395(10223): e30–1.

15. Sheahan TP, Sims AC, Leist SR, *et al.* Comparative therapeutic efficacy of remdesivir and combination lopinavir, ritonavir, and interferon beta against MERS-CoV. *Nat Commun.* 2020;11(1):222.

16. Shen K, Yang Y, Wang T, *et al.* Diagnosis, treatment, and prevention of 2019 novel coronavirus infection in children: Experts' consensus statement. *World J Pediatr.* Published Feb 7, 2020. https://doi.org/10.1007/s12519-020-00343-7.

17. Shi Y, Gao J-H, Wang L-S. Perinatal and neonatal management plan for prevention and control of SARS-CoV-2 infection (1st Edition). [Chinese]. *Chin J Contemp Pediatr.* 2020;22(2):87–90.

18. Vincent MJ, Bergeron E, Benjannet S, *et al.* Chloroquine is a potent inhibitor of SARS coronavirus infection and spread. *Virol J.* 2005;2:69.

19. Wang M, Cao R, Zhang L, *et al.* Remdesivir and chloroquine effectively inhibit the recently emerged novel coronavirus (2019-nCoV) *in vitro. Cell Res.* 2020;30:269–71.

20. Zhao Y, Zou L, Wang L, Wang Z. Advice on the administration of pregnant women with 2019-nCoV infection (2nd Edition). http://guide.medlive.cn/guideline/19866. Published Jan 28, 2020. Accessed Feb 20, 2020.

21. Zumla A, Chan JFW, Azhar EI, Hui DSC, Yuen K-Y. Coronaviruses — drug discovery and therapeutic options. *Nat Rev Drug Discov.* 2016;15(5):327–47.

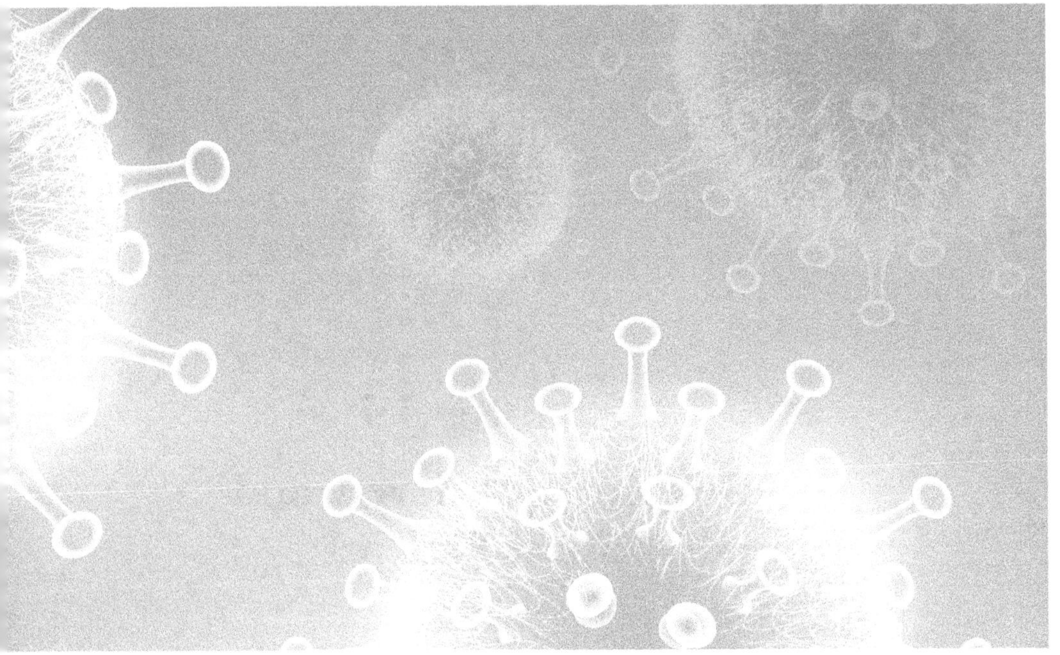

Part 7

Treatment of Severe and Critical Patients

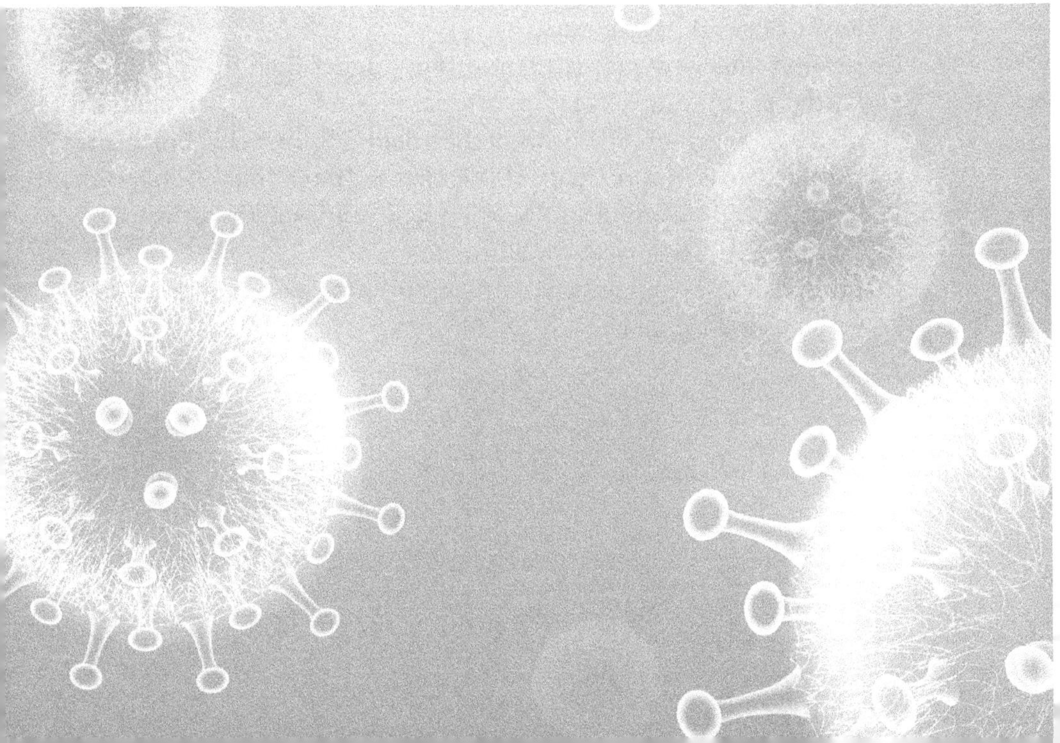

Chapter 19
Definition of Severe and Critical Patients

Based on the *"Diagnosis and Treatment Protocol for Novel Coronavirus Pneumonia (Trial Version 6)"* by the National Health Commission of China:

19.1 Serious Patients Match at Least One of the Following

(1) Patients have difficulty breathing, with a breath frequency no lower than 30 per minute;

(2) Resting finger oxygen saturation is no higher than 93%;

(3) Partial pressure of oxygen in arterial blood (P_aO_2) / fraction of inhaled oxygen (FiO_2) is no higher than 300 mmHg. For high-altitude areas (more than 1000 meters (0.62 mile) above sea level), use the formula P_aO_2 / FiO_2 × (atmospheric pressure / 760 mmHg) to correct for altitude;

(4) Lung radiology suggests more than 50% progression of the lesion within 24–48 hours.

19.2 Critical Patients Match at Least One of the Following

(1) Patients exhibit respiratory failure and needs mechanical ventilation;
(2) Patients go into shock;
(3) Patients have other organ failure and need monitoring and treatment in ICU.

Chapter 20
Comprehensive Treatment
of Severe and Critical Patients

COVID-19 is not just pneumonia. Treating serious patients calls for the integration of multiple subjects, which has become a highlight of the treatment.

During treatment, the departments of infectious diseases, respiration, and traditional Chinese medicine (TCM) play important roles when mild patients progress to serious cases. It is also indispensable to have multi-organ function maintenance from intensive care medicine, airway management from critical respiratory illness and respiratory therapists, critical support from extracorporeal membrane oxygenation (ECMO, also known as artificial lung), filtration of inflammation factors from the department of nephrology, treatment of cardiac arrhythmia from department of cardiology, rapid intubation from department of anesthesiology, accurate anti-infective treatment from departments of infectious diseases and clinical microbiology, as well as personalized treatment from department of TCM.

Most of the extremely critical patients need mechanical ventilation; some of them were supported with ECMO. Nonetheless, we found that in addition to damage to the respiratory system, serious patients often had damage in multiple organs and systems, including the heart, kidneys, and blood coagulation system in the early stages of the disease, some even before hospital admission. Therefore, in addition to respiratory support, systemic multi-organ support is critical.

Once the condition has progressed to critical (needing mechanical ventilation), the prognosis is significantly worse. From this perspective, it is crucial to have a comprehensive multi-department treatment plan to prevent mild patients from progressing to seriously ill.

This disease by nature is a systemic one, and it is appropriate to name it coronavirus disease from a treatment perspective as well. The Shanghai expert team's cumulative experience in treating COVID-19 patients has been used to form a consensus on how to comprehensively treat the disease. Details of this consensus are found in the Appendix.

Chapter 21
Treatment of Severe and Critical Patients

21.1 Warning Indicators of Clinical Deterioration

Severe COVID-19 patients require close monitoring of vital signs, which consist of heart rate, blood pressure, peripheral capillary oxygen saturation (SpO_2), respiratory rate, and state of consciousness. Regular laboratory tests and imaging examinations should be performed, including complete blood count, urinalysis, blood biochemistry (liver and kidney function, lactate, blood glucose, and electrolytes), lactate dehydrogenase (LDH), cardiac markers, C-reactive protein (CRP), procalcitonin (PCT), coagulation test, arterial blood gas, electrocardiography (ECG) and chest imaging.

Clinical deterioration should be considered when the following situations emerge:

(1) Peripheral lymphocyte count progressively decreases;
(2) Peripheral inflammatory factor levels gradually increase;
(3) Lactate that indicates tissue oxygenation continues to climb;
(4) Pulmonary lesions on high-resolution computed tomography (HRCT) expand rapidly.

21.2 Treatment Principles

In addition to supportive care interventions, proactive measures should be adopted to prevent and manage complications of COVID-19 and secondary infections. Good control of underlying medical conditions should be ensured and timely organ function support should be provided when needed.

21.3 Oxygen Therapy and Respiratory Support

In the *Guidelines on Severe and Critical COVID-19 Diagnosis and Treatment* (2nd trial edition-issued by China's National Health Commission, oxygen therapy includes oxygen administration via nasal cannula or face shields, high flow nasal cannula (HFNC), noninvasive ventilation (NIV), invasive mechanical ventilation and extracorporeal membrane oxygenation (ECMO). It emphasizes that patients on either HFNC or NIV should be closely monitored for two hours, and endotracheal intubation and invasive ventilation should be implemented without delay if the patient's condition does not improve or HFNC/NIV is not tolerated. "Lung protective ventilation" strategy for invasive mechanical ventilation ought to be adopted. For patients with severe acute respiratory distress syndrome (ARDS), prone positioning ventilation is recommended. Extracorporeal membrane oxygenation (ECMO) should be considered if mechanical ventilation fails. Since no specific parameter has been recommended for clinical practice, expert consensus on respiratory therapy procedure in severe COVID-19 published in February 2020 first introduced oxygenation index to classify severe cases into three groups: mild, mild–moderate, and moderate–severe. Physicians should choose appropriate ventilatory support strategy according to the disease severity.

21.3.1 *Ventilatory support in mild ARDS*
(200 mmHg ≤ PaO$_2$/FiO$_2$ < 300 mmHg)

HFNC is preferred on 40–50 L/min and FiO$_2$ 100%. Patients' vital signs and oxygenation should be closely monitored in case of worsening respiratory status. Previous studies showed that patients receiving HFNC with higher oxygen requirement tended to fail with NIV. In addition, delayed invasive mechanical ventilation was associated with increased mortality. So, we recommend early endotracheal intubation and invasive mechanical ventilation once the patients' conditions do not improve or HFNC/NIV is not tolerated.

21.3.2 *Ventilatory support in mild–moderate ARDS (150 mmHg ≤ PaO_2/FiO_2 <200 mmHg)*

Given its high failure rate, NIV with close monitoring is optional. The initial NIV parameters are to be set as follows: inspiratory positive airway pressure (IPAP) 8–10 cmH_2O (1 cmH_2O = 0.098 kPa), expiratory positive airway pressure (EPAP) 5–8 cmH_2O, FiO_2 100%. Experts recommend that after a two-hour trial, if tidal volume (Vt) ≤ 9 ml/kg, continue NIV; if Vt > 12 ml/kg, stop NIV immediately and switch to endotracheal intubation and invasive ventilation. For those with Vt 9–12 ml/kg, apply NIV for another six hours; if Vt ≤ 9 ml/kg, continue NIV; otherwise escalate to intubation and invasive mechanical ventilation.

21.3.3 *Ventilatory support in moderate–severe ARDS (PaO_2/FiO_2 < 150 mmHg)*

Invasive mechanical ventilation should be performed with "lung protective ventilation" strategy to minimize ventilator-induced lung injury, which is low tidal volume (4–6 ml/kg ideal body weight, IBW) and static inspiratory pressure (plateau pressure < 30 cmH_2O). Start with a tidal volume of 6 ml/kg IBW and monitor inspiratory plateau pressure. If plateau pressure > 30 cmH_2O, decrease Vt by 1 ml/kg until inspiratory plateau pressure < 30 cmH_2O or Vt = 4 ml/kg, while minute ventilation should be ensured by increasing respiratory rate to prevent CO_2 retention.

When the patient is recovering with inspiratory plateau pressure < 30 cmH_2O, FiO_2 ≤ 40% and PEEP ≤ 5 cmH_2O, select pressure support ventilation instead of a mandatory mode. Weaning from invasive ventilation can be considered only if all of the listed criteria are met:

(1) Being conscious and responsive;
(2) Hemodynamic stability, that is, no vasoactive agents use, or dopamine dose less than 5 µg/(kg·min), or dopamine dose less than 20 µg/min;
(3) With low level of invasive ventilatory support (pressure support ventilation, $FiO_2 \leq 40\%$, PEEP ≤ 5 cmH_2O), $SpO_2 > 95\%$ or $PaO_2/FiO_2 \geq 250$ mmHg, 35 mmHg $\leq$ partial pressure of carbon dioxide in arterial blood ($PaCO_2$) ≤ 50 mmHg, or rapid shallow breathing index [RR/Vt (L)] ≤ 105.

Spontaneous breathing trial (SBT) is recommended before extubation.

21.3.4 *Prone positioning ventilation*

Prone positioning ventilation for more than 12 hours per day is recommended if $PaO_2/FiO_2 < 150$ mmHg persists. Prone positioning theoretically recruits the collapsed gravity-dependent lung regions and optimizes ventilation–perfusion matching, leading to improved oxygenation in severe COVID-19 patients.

21.4 Extracorporeal Membrane Oxygenation

ECMO, known as extracorporeal life support system (ECLS), provides prolonged cardiac and respiratory support for critically ill patients with refractory circulatory, respiratory failure, or both. This technology has been increasingly used in the recent decade. ARDS, a common indication for ECMO, is ameliorated through gas exchange by means of an extracorporeal membrane instead of alveoli. ECMO may facilitate "lung protective ventilation" and "lung rest" strategies to promote recovery. According to *Guidelines on COVID-19 Diagnosis and Treatment (6ᵗʰ trial edition)* issued by China's National Health Commission, ECMO should be indicated as a rescue therapy when the conventional therapy fails in critical patients affected by

COVID-19. However, as a resource-intensive form of life support, ECMO's role in the management of COVID-19 is unclear at this point. An article published by the *Journal of the American Medical Association* (*JAMA*) stated that both patients' conditions and medical resource availability should be considered before starting an ECMO program. Ensuring wide availability of oxygen and pulse oximetry is much more crucial for saving lives in a pandemic.

21.4.1 *Timing of starting ECMO*

For critical COVID-19 patients with refractory hypoxemia despite standard lung protective ventilation and prone positioning, ECMO should be started prior to hypoxia-induced multiorgan injuries and mechanical ventilation at high settings. Under optimal ventilation conditions ($FiO_2 \geq 80\%$, $Vt = 6$ ml/kg IBW, $PEEP \geq 10$ cmH_2O), ECMO can be started if one of the following criteria is met without contraindications:

(1) $PaO_2/FiO_2 < 50$ mmHg for more than three hours;
(2) $PaO_2/FiO_2 < 80$ mmHg for more than six hours;
(3) $FiO_2 = 1.0$, $PaO_2/FiO_2 < 100$ mmHg;
(4) Arterial blood pH < 7.25 and $PaCO_2 > 60$ mmHg for more than six hours, combined with respiratory rate > 35 breaths/min;
(5) Respiratory rate >35 breaths/min, arterial blood pH < 7.2 and plateau pressure > 30 cmH_2O;
(6) Severe air leak syndrome;
(7) Combined with cardiogenic shock or cardiac arrest.

21.4.2 *Contraindications*

There are no absolute contraindications to ECMO. However, certain conditions that are associated with a poor outcome despite ECMO can be considered as relative contraindications:

(1) Nonrecoverable comorbidity;
(2) High risk of systemic bleeding that is contraindicated to anticoagulation;

(3) Mechanical ventilation at high settings ($FiO_2 > 90\%$, plateau pressure > 30 cmH$_2$O) for more than seven days;
(4) No specific age contraindication but higher risk of death as age increases;
(5) Multiple organ failure;
(6) Moderate–severe aortic insufficiency and acute aortic dissection should also be considered as contraindicators in case of veno–arterial extracorporeal membrane oxygenation (VA–ECMO) for cardiac support;
(7) Immunosuppression (absolute neutrophil count $< 0.4 \times 10^9$/L);
(8) Limited vascular access due to malformations or disease of large peripheral blood vessels.

21.4.3 *Modalities*

ECMO has two main configurations depending on its purpose: veno–venous extracorporeal membrane oxygenation (VV–ECMO) and veno–arterial extracorporeal membrane oxygenation (VA–ECMO).

(1) VV–ECMO is preferred when cardiac function is adequate. Normally VV access is by femoral and jugular veins, draining blood from the vena cava to the oxygenator where oxygenation occurs.
(2) VA–ECMO is preferred for respiratory failure combined with cardiogenic shock or decompensated heart failure, when cardiac support and respiratory support are both required. Usually VA access is by the femoral vein and artery. Veno–arterial–venous extracorporeal membrane oxygenation (VAV–ECMO), which adds a second supplying cannula into the right internal jugular vein, may be used to supplement upper body oxygenation in case of differential hypoxia.

21.5 Hemodynamic Management

It is important to choose easy and feasible hemodynamic monitoring techniques (i.e., echocardiography) to monitor the circulation intensively. It is critical to determine the type of shock in hemodynamically unstable patients, for instance, whether it is septic shock due to the presence of fever or cardiogenic shock caused by cardiac disfunction.

The most appropriate therapy should be selected to reverse the etiology, with the aim of correcting tissue hypoperfusion and delivering adequate oxygen.

21.6 Continuous Renal Replacement Therapy

The incidence of acute kidney injury (AKI) in COVID-19 patients ranges from 3% to 10%. In addition, life-threatening complications including systemic inflammatory response syndrome (SIRS) and multiple organ dysfunction syndrome (MODS) may also occur in severe cases. In the *Guidelines on COVID-19 Diagnosis and Treatment* (6th trial edition) issued by China's National Health Commission, blood purification is recommended for critically ill patients with overactive inflammatory response. Continuous renal replacement therapy (CRRT) in COVID-19 is designed to maintain electrolyte and acid-base homeostasis, remove excess metabolic products, and alleviate fluid overload. The appropriate use of CRRT provides advanced life support and plays a role in reducing COVID-19 fatality rate.

21.6.1 *Indications*

(1) Severe inflammatory response due to MODS, sepsis, septic shock, ARDS, etc;
(2) Severe volume overload, life-threatening electrolyte and acid-base abnormalities;
(3) AKI requiring blood purification;
(4) COVID-19 patients requiring maintenance hemodialysis;
(5) COVID-19 patients with existing severe acute pancreatitis or chronic heart failure.

21.6.2 *Contraindications*

There are no absolute contraindications to CRRT. But attention needs to be paid to CRRT if the following conditions exist:

(1) Inability to establish vascular access;
(2) Refractory hypotension.

21.6.3 *Modalities*

(1) Both continuous veno–venous hemofiltration (CVVH) and continuous veno–venous hemodiafiltration (CVVHDF) could be used when dealing with severe pH or electrolyte disorder. The dose of renal replacement therapy (RRT) should be prescribed according to the severity of the disease and actual achievement of goals.

(2) The indication of slow continuous ultrafiltration (SCUF) is fluid overload without uremia or significant electrolyte imbalance. The ultrafiltration rates of 2–5 ml/min are preferred, which can be adjusted according to clinical situations. Typically, the ultrafiltration volume should not exceed 4 liters in a single treatment.

(3) CVVH, continuous plasma filtration absorption (CPFA), or both are recommended to relieve inflammatory cascade. Hemoperfusion can also be administered if needed.

(4) ECMO could also be adopted in treating severe ARDS.

21.6.4 *Anticoagulation*

Physicians should base the decision to use anticoagulation for CRRT on the assessment of the patient's coagulation and contraindications to anticoagulants. The contraindications for regional citrate anticoagulation include $PaO_2 < 60$ mmHg and/or tissue hypoperfusion (blood lactate > 4 mmol/L), metabolic alkalosis, hypernatremia, and severe liver failure. Severe liver failure is also the contraindication to argatroban. For patients with a history of allergy reaction to heparin or heparin–induced thrombocytopenia (HIT), unfractionated and low-molecular-weight heparin must be stopped. However, for patients without an increased bleeding risk or impaired coagulation, or in a hypercoagulable state, we recommend using either unfractionated or low-molecular-weight heparin. For patients with active bleeding or increased bleeding risk, we suggest performing CRRT without anticoagulation if international normalized ratio (INR) is more than or equal to 1.5. If INR < 1.5, use a standard protocol of regional citrate anticoagulation in a patient without contraindications for citrate; otherwise, choose argatroban if allowed. For patients with disseminated intravascular coagulation (DIC), based on supplementary coagulation factors administration and primary anticoagulation with heparin, we suggest performing CRRT without anticoagulation if INR $\geq$ 1.5; otherwise increase the dose of heparins properly.

21.7 Nutritional Support

For severe COVID-19 patients, early nutrition should be started as soon as hemodynamics is stable with fluid resuscitation. Either gastric or jejunal feeding can be performed. The feeding target should be 25–30 kcal/(kg·d) by starting with a low dose in a diluted concentration. Continuous enteral nutrition rather than bolus is preferred. For critical illness, a higher protein intake, 1.3–2.0 g/kg protein per day, should be delivered progressively, and supplemented with protein powder to achieve the goal if necessary. Enteral nutrition enriched with ω-3 fatty acid can be administered. Parenteral lipid emulsions enriched with eicosapentaenoic acid (EPA) and docosahexaenoic acid (DHA) can be provided for patients receiving parenteral nutrition.

Chapter 22
Precautions for the Treatment of Severe Patients

22.1 Glucocorticoids

Glucocorticoids are considered to be able to inhibit excessive inflammatory response, cell proliferation, and collagen deposition. However, its effects on mortality and outcomes in acute respiratory distress syndrome (ARDS) and severe viral pneumonia remain controversial.

Previous studies have shown that the glucocorticoid therapy in SARS was associated with poorer outcomes, higher rate of ICU admission, and increased mortality. In patients with MERS, corticosteroids did not contribute to any difference in mortality, but MERS coronavirus RNA clearance was delayed. Available evidence cannot support the use of corticosteroids as standard care for patients with severe influenza. Only patients with community-acquired pneumonia may benefit from the short-term treatment with corticosteroids, by reducing the risk of ARDS and shortening the course of the disease.

Except for clinical trials, routine use of systemic corticosteroids for treatment of viral pneumonia or ARDS is not recommended by the World Health Organization (WHO) in treating COVID-19 critical cases. As of February 2020, China's National Health Commission has updated six editions of *Guidelines on COVID-19 Diagnosis and Treatment*. All plans recommended that corticosteroids administration in severe and critically ill patients with COVID-19 should depend on the severity of dyspnea and the change in chest imaging. Treatment with glucocorticoids should not exceed 1–2 mg/(kg·d) methylprednisolone or equivalents for three to five days. So far, no valid evidence has confirmed the value of glucocorticoids in the treatment of COVID-19, and results of further randomized controlled trials are being anticipated.

22.2 Immunotherapy

22.2.1 *Intravenous immunoglobulin*

At present, there is insufficient evidence of intravenous immunoglobulin (IVIG) efficacy against COVID-19. Severe and critical patients with COVID-19 could use IVIG based on their conditions.

22.2.2 *Convalescent plasma*

Convalescent plasma (CP), obtained from a patient who has survived a previous infection, is a source of specific antibody to neutralize the pathogen. According to previous studies, CP is considered a potential therapy for emerging infectious diseases such as SARS and MERS. However, data on the efficacy and safety of convalescent plasma in COVID-19 are limited, and more scientific experiments and clinical trials are needed.

For severe and critically ill COVID-19 patients whose conditions continue to deteriorate, CP can be used as a specific anti-SARS-CoV-2 treatment. Pre-transfusion measurement of neutralizing antibody titers should be performed and neutralizing antibody titers of at least 1:160 is recommended. The dose of CP depends on the patient's condition and body weight. Typically, 200–500 ml (i.e., 4–5 ml/kg) CP are infused in two settings.

22.3 Targeted Antimicrobial Therapy Against Secondary Bacterial and Fungal Infection

22.3.1 *Pathogen detection*

Microbial monitoring should be performed in all severe and critically ill patients with COVID-19. It is required to collect sputum and urine specimens for routine cultures, and collect blood cultures promptly if patients develop high fever. For patients with suspected sepsis who have intravascular access devices, two sets of blood cultures should be drawn at the same time, with one from peripheral sites and the other from the catheters. Also, molecular diagnosis for pathogen identification in peripheral blood could be considered, including PCR-based molecular biological techniques and metagenomics next generation sequencing (mNGS) tests.

22.3.2 *The value of inflammatory biomarkers*

High PCT levels are of clinical significance in the diagnosis of sepsis and septic shock. CRP is less specific in bacterial and fungal infections, though it also increases in response to clinical deterioration.

22.3.3 *Antimicrobial therapy*

Critical patients intubated or with a tracheotomy are especially vulnerable to secondary bacterial and fungal infections at later stages. Empirical administration of antimicrobials should be initiated as soon as possible after identification of sepsis. Before pathogen evidence is established, combined therapy with broad-spectrum antimicrobials is recommended for patients presenting septic shock to cover the most likely pathogens, including Enterobacteriaceae, Staphylococcus, and Enterococcus. Fungal coverage should also be considered since invasive candidiasis is more common in critically ill patients. Prolonged hospital stay of severe cases probably leads to the development of antimicrobial resistance, so antimicrobial therapy should be adjusted according to the antimicrobial susceptibility testing results.

22.4 Criteria for Discharge from ICU

When a patient's physiologic status has stabilized and oxygenation has improved without a need for life support, the patient should be discharged from ICU as soon as possible. All of the discharge criteria should be met as follows:

(1) Conscious patients who are able to obey instructions and stop using sedatives, analgesics, and neuromuscular blockers;

(2) Successful weaning from mechanical ventilation, respiratory rate < 30 breaths/min and SpO_2 > 93% on room air or low-flow oxygen therapy (via nasal cannula or simple face mask);

(3) Hemodynamically stable without vasopressors or fluid resuscitation;

(4) No other acute or progressive organ dysfunction that requires supportive care such as blood purification.

References

1. Du B, Qiu HB, Zhan X, *et al*. Pharmacotherapeutics for the New Coronavirus Pneumonia. *Zhonghua Jie He He Hu Xi Za Zhi*. 2020;43(3):173–176.

2. Expert consensus on application of CRRT in treatment of Novel Coronavirus Pneumonia. National Center for Nephrology Medical Quality Management and Control, Blood Purification Therapy and Engineering Technology Society of China International Exchange and Promotion Association for Medical and Healthcare, Committee of Blood Purification Therapy of the PLA. (2020-02-06) [2020-02-23]. http://www.cnrds.net/Static/file/新型冠状病毒肺炎救治中CRRT应用的专家意见%2020200206.pdf.

3. A circular on issuing Guidelines on COVID-19 Diagnosis and Treatment (6th provisional edition). National Health Commission, Office of National Administration of Traditional Chinese Medicine. (2020-02-18) [2020-02-23]. http://www.nhc.gov.cn/yzygj/s7653p/202002/8334a8326dd94d329df351d7da8aefc2.shtml.

4. A circular on issuing Guidelines on Severe and Critical COVID-19 Diagnosis and Treatment (2nd provisional edition). National Health Commission. (2020-02-14) [2020-02-23].

5. Zheng RQ, Hu M, Li XY, *et al*. Expert consensus on respiratory therapy procedure in severe COVID-19. *Chin J Crit Care Intensive Care Med*. 2020;06(2020-02-09) [2020-02-23]. http://rs.yiigle.com/resource_static.jspx? contentId=1180124.

6. Chinese Society of Extracorporeal Life Support of Chinese Medical Doctor Association. Expert consensus on the timing and modalities of extracorporeal life support in critically ill patients with COVID-19. *Chin J Crit Care Intensive Care Med*. 2020;06(2020-02-09) [2020-02-23]. http://rs.yiigle.com/resource_static.jspx? contentId=1180131.

7. Special Expert Group for Control of the Epidemic of Novel Coronavirus Pneumonia of the Chinese Preventive Medicine Association. An update on the epidemiological characteristics of novel coronavirus pneumonia (COVID-19). *Zhonghua Liu Xing Bing Xue Za Zhi* 2020; 41(2):139–144.

8. Annane D, Renault A, Brun-Buisson C, *et al*. Hydrocortisone plus fludrocortisone for adults with septic shock. *N Engl J Med.* 2018;378(9):809–818.

9. Arabi YM, Mandourah Y, Al-Hameed F, *et al*. Corticosteroid therapy for critically ill patients with Middle Ease respiratory syndrome. *Am J Respir Crit Care Med.* 2018; 197(6):757–767.

10. Chen N, Zhou M, Dong X, *et al*. Epidemiological and clinical characteristics of 99 cases of 2019 novel coronavirus pneumonia in Wuhan, China: A descriptive study. *Lancet.* 2020;395(10223):507–513.

11. Kovacs JA, Masur H. Evolving health effects of pneumocystis: One hundred years of progress in diagnosis and treatment. JAMA 2009; 301(24):2578–2585.

12. Mair-Jenkins J, Saavedra-Campos M, Baillie JK, *et al*. The effectiveness of convalescent plasma and hyperimmune immunoglobulin for the treatment of severe acute respiratory infections of viral etiology: A systematic review and exploratory meta-analysis. *J Infect Dis* 2015; 211(1):80-90.

13. Marano G, Vaglio S, Pupella S, *et al*. Convalescent plasma: New evidence for an old therapeutic tool? *Blood Transfus.* 2016;14(2):152–157.

14. Ni YN, Chen G, Sun J, Liang BM, Liang ZA. The effect of corticosteroids on mortality of patients with influenza pneumonia: A systematic review and meta-analysis. *Crit Care.* 2019;23(1):99.

15. Stockman LJ, Bellamy R, Garner P. SARS: Systematic review of treatment effects. *PLoS Med.* 2006;3(9): e343.

16. Venkatesh B, Finfer S, Cohen J, *et al*. Adjunctive glucocorticoid therapy in patients with septic shock. *N Engl J Med.* 2018;378(9):797–808.

17. Wan YD, Sun TW, Liu ZQ, Zhang SG, Wang LX, Kan QC. Efficacy and safety of corticosteroids for community-acquired pneumonia: A systematic review and meta-analysis. *Chest.* 2016;149(1):209–219.

18. World Health Organization. Clinical management of severe acute respiratory infection when novel coronavirus (nCoV) infection is suspected: interim guidance. (2020-01-28) [2020-02-23]. http://www.who.int/publications-detail/clinical-managemeng-of-severe-acute-respiratory-infection-when-novel-coronavirus-(ncov)-infection-is-suspected.

19. Zhang Y, Sun W, Svendsen ER, *et al*. Do corticosteroids reduce the mortality of influenza A (H1N1) infection? A meta-analysis. *Crit Care.* 2015;19:46.

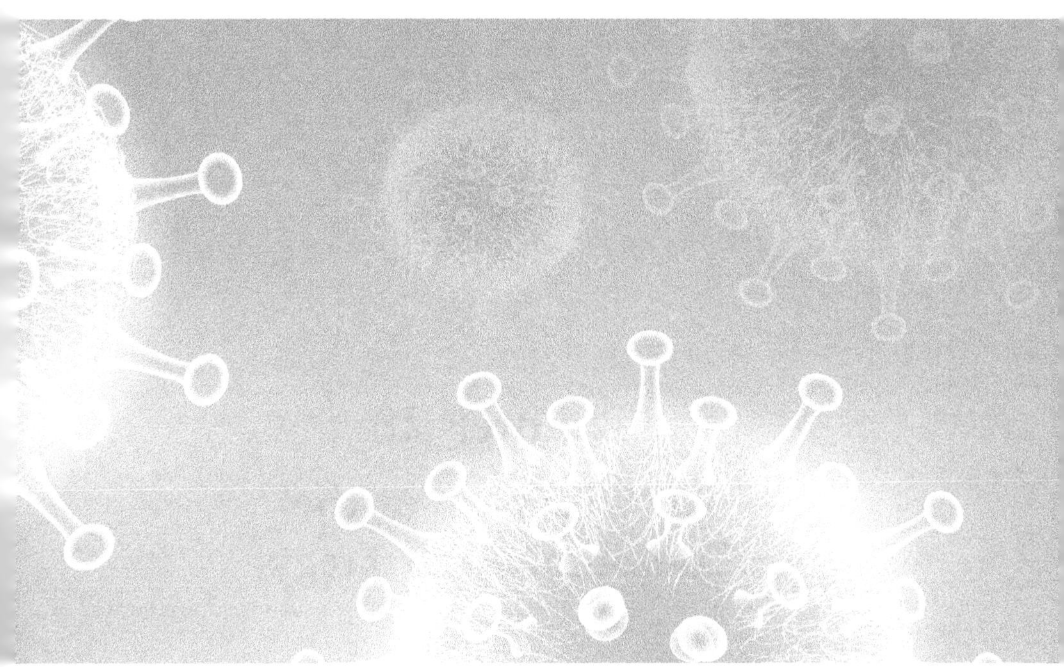

Part 8

Containment Strategy and Prevention and Control of Nosocomial Infection

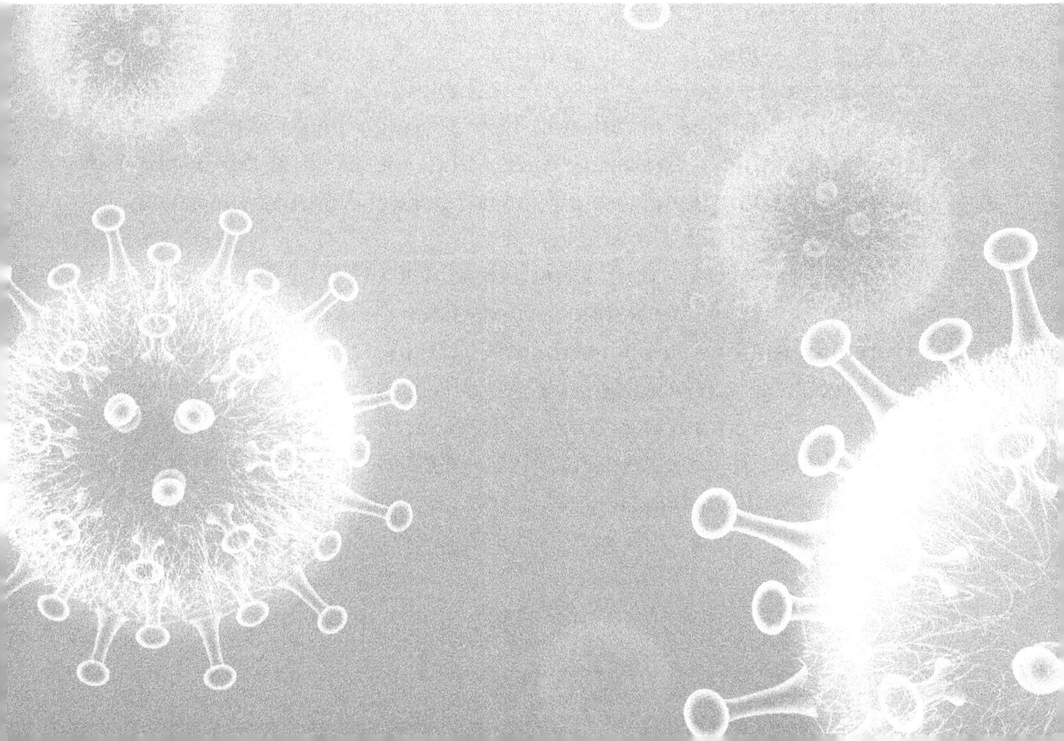

Chapter 23
An Overview of the Containment Strategy

As the guiding principle to control and prevent influenza pandemic, the containment strategy proposed by the World Health Organization (WHO) refers to the adoption of multilevel medical and non-medical interventions limited to certain geographical regions in different stages of the flu pandemic in order to rapidly cut off the spread of the disease.

In December 2019, COVID-19 broke out in the city of Wuhan in Hubei province and immediately swept across China. In response to the epidemic, China's government employed the containment strategy to control further transmission. A series of core measures including social mobilization, strengthening case isolation, close contact tracing, curbing population flow through lockdown of affected areas and traffic restrictions, increasing social distance, improving environmental hygiene, and enhancing personal protection have been implemented, which showed results.

Based on the current knowledge of COVID-19 and concerns over the Spring Festival travel rush, China's government raised its emergency response level in January 2020 in a comprehensive way. At state level, a group leading novel coronavirus prevention and control was set up, with joint prevention and control mechanism established. National Health Commission (NHC) of China has managed COVID-19 with measures typically used for category-A infectious diseases even though it was classified as a category-B infectious disease, and treated it as an internationally quarantinable infectious disease. Thirty-one provinces, autonomous regions, and municipalities directly under the Central Government in mainland China activated first-level public health emergency response. Meanwhile, containment measures have been imposed on seriously affected areas including Wuhan in order to confine the disease to limited areas and prevent it from further transmission to other parts of China and abroad.

The containment measures include: (1) reducing the flow of people and preventing virus spread through lockdown of affected areas and traffic restrictions; (2) strengthening the detection, isolation, and treatment of cases, and close contact tracing to ensure early identification and effective control of the infection source; (3) cancelling mass gatherings, postponing reopening of schools and resumption of work, extending the Chinese New Year holiday, and increasing social distance to reduce susceptible people's contact with and exposure to the infected; (4) improving the hygiene, disinfection, and ventilation of public transport and public areas to cut off transmission routes; (5) implementing pre-examination and triage of contagious disease in medical institutions, tightening regulations on visiting hospital, and ensuring medical staff's self-protection to avoid nosocomial cross infection; and (6) promoting hygiene by calling on people to take self-protective measures including wearing masks, following respiratory etiquette instructions, and keeping hands clean to protect the susceptible population.

Gauging the effectiveness of containment also requires objective evaluation indicators. It is critical to assess the result of containment measures from the perspective of public health strategy, with consideration of actual situations. As one model-based research indicated, traffic restrictions imposed on various parts of China could slow down the spread of SARS-CoV-2 from Wuhan to the rest of the country by 2.9 days. Another research found measures taken in the early stage like isolating cases and increasing social distance proved effective in keeping the disease from spreading widely within a short time. On the whole, containment measures have to some degree reduced the risk of continuous spread of the virus in communities outside Wuhan in China. By delaying the peak period of the epidemic, they have alleviated the burden on medical resources and gained precious time to prepare for a possible global pandemic. Nevertheless, they have also unavoidably exerted negative impact on people's life and social production in worst virus-hit areas including Wuhan, leading to huge losses in economy and society.

Chapter 24
Preventive Measures

Clinically speaking, there are not many targeted and specific treatments for COVID-19; it is mainly treated through supportive and symptomatic therapies. Therefore, for such virus-induced disease, precaution is far more important than cure. Prevention does not only refer to wearing personal protective equipment, which is the most basic precaution, but also requires higher level of prevention including environmental control and administration. Environmental control means setting up special areas or wards that can isolate air and droplets, establishing biosafety laboratory, and installing biosafety equipment. It also means reasonable layout and procedure as well as reasonable section division and entrance design for reducing human contact. The highest level of administration is defined as a series of procedure control systems including pre-examination and triage system; fever clinic system; prevention, control, and emergence response system; risk-based treatment system; and personal protective equipment storage system. These are used for eliminating risk exposure as early as possible. This chapter discusses specific measures to prevent SARS-CoV-2 infection based on the three steps of stopping epidemic spread: infection source control, transmission route cutoff, and protection of susceptible population.

24.1 Control of Infection Source

The major infection source of COVID-19 is those who are infected with SARS-CoV-2 and possibly asymptomatic cases. Up to now, asymptomatic cases mainly found among close contacts are either those not yet sick or those asymptomatically infected. Therefore, infection source control means early detection and diagnosis, with different levels of isolation and observation to prevent further transmission of the disease.

24.1.1. *Setup of fever clinics in hospitals to accelerate the diagnosis of suspected cases*

Medical institutions should set up independent fever clinics where central air-conditioning is shut off or independent ventilation system is installed. Disinfection and isolation should be standardized and proper preventative measures ought to be taken to protect medical staff. Any suspected case needs isolation in single room. For those who remain suspected cases after the consultation of hospital experts and attending physicians, direct online report of them should be delivered in two hours and their samples should be collected for nucleic acid testing. The diagnostic process of infection ought to be simplified as much as possible, exercised as early as possible and down to the community level so as to shorten the time for diagnosis or exclusion. Currently, confirmed cases are decided upon the evidence that the detection is positive for SARS-CoV-2 nucleic acid by real-time RT-PCR, or genome sequence of the virus is very close to that of SARS-CoV-2. There have been reports saying SARS-CoV-2 IgM Antibody Test Kit with the adoption of immune colloidal gold technique is expected to deliver test results observed by naked eyes within 15 minutes, which will significantly shorten test time and overcome the constraints of technical staff and location. However, its diagnostic value still needs further investigation and proof.

24.1.2 *Isolation and classified treatment of confirmed cases based on the level of infection severity*

Independent isolation wards need to be set up to receive and treat patients with confirmed infection and they should be located far away from the downtown area if conditions permit. Confirmed cases should be classified on the level of their infection severity. Severe or critical patients and other pneumonia patients must be isolated and should receive treatment in designated hospitals with good conditions for isolation and protection. Suspected cases are supposed to be in single room isolation while confirmed cases could be gathered and treated in the same ward. Asymptomatic cases and patients with mild symptoms only need syptomatic treatment and do not require special treatment. However, it is important to isolate and observe their conditions by converting stadiums, schools, and hotels into temporary treatment centers for concentrated management (like Fangcang shelter hospital in Wuhan). These facilities are equipped with medical staff making regular medical inspections on patients, and seek to reduce the occupation of limited beds in hospitals. During isolation, if patients get worse, they will be transferred to designated hospitals for treatment. Patients who are allowed to leave hospital must be in strict accordance with the standards for the discharge of confirmed cases from hospital.

24.1.3 *Management of close contacts*

When there are patients confirmed with COVID-19, departments for disease control and prevention should make prompt investigations of people around confirmed cases and carry out thorough disinfection of places where they have been. Since asymptomatic cases make up a proportion of close contacts, tracing of close contacts and screening for infection must be strengthened. If conditions allow, samples ought to be collected for testing as soon as close contacts are found and etiological examination should be conducted when they are discharged from medical observation. If conditions do not permit, medical observation measures are supposed to be taken with a time span of two weeks to prevent further spread of the potential source of infection. A few reports also claimed that the longest incubation period of the virus could be more than two weeks but whether it is necessary to prolong the time for observation requires more data for discussion. If anyone in a group of people under quarantine is confirmed with infection during concentrated observation, the rest needs to go through one more incubation period of medical observation from the day when the last case was confirmed.

24.1.4 *Enhanced community management*

Community is the frontline of joint prevention and control of the outbreak. Digital management for a matrix of urban communities in a thorough way is crucial to make sure all measures of prevention and control are put in place. With a special focus on tracing key groups, communities are required to release health tips, promote and disseminate knowledge of COVID-19, and guide ordinary people to do self-protection, voluntary report, and cooperation in health screening. Screening spots for prevention and control need to be set up in transportation of road, railway, air, and water, as well as in public workplaces to monitor the population.

24.2   Cutoff of Transmission Routes

Respiratory droplets and close unprotected contacts are the main routes of transmission. Transmission through aerosols is possible in the case of long-term exposure to high-concentration aerosols in a relatively closed environment. Precautions need be taken by hospitals, communities, public places, and individuals to cut off the routes of transmission.

24.2.1 *Hospital measures*

Great importance should be attached to disinfection and isolation. Through cooperation between different departments, hospitals are supposed to make sure disinfection measures are implemented with strict standards and effective results.

The diagnosis and treatment sections need to be managed with strengthened efforts with screening carried out in fever clinics and quarantine wards. The key section for diagnosis and treatment should be designed with "three areas and two entrances". Three areas include clean area, potentially contaminated area (originally called partially contaminated area or buffer area) and contaminated area; two entrances refer to the entrance for patients and the entrance for medical staff. Between clean area, potentially contaminated area, and contaminated area, there should be substantial physical barriers. Such design aimed at reducing cross infection between medical staff and patients, as well as between flow of people and goods, represents the most important and fundamental measure for epidemic prevention and control. These sections are relatively independent and well-ventilated with appropriate physical separation. Medical staff need to know which level of medical equipment to wear in certain areas and avoid crossing areas without permission, which could lead to dangerous risk exposure.

Medical staff should adopt scientific and proper self-protective measures and choose suitable protective equipment for different positions. During the pandemic, it is important to minimize meaningless upgrade of protective equipment since global personal protective equipment (PPE) is in short supply. Training should be targeted at medical staff in different positions to enable them to familiarise with PPE use.

Medical staff should be reasonably deployed and should not be exposed to isolation area for too long. The number of staff working in an isolation area could be reduced by letting staff outside the isolation area help finish up some of their colleagues' work through video call or other online technologies. Medical workers cannot work continuously and intensively for too long, and adequate time for rest should be guaranteed through regular shifts.

Management on outpatient clinic procedure and hospital visits ought to be strengthened. Medical institutions should define the procedure and set up contingency plan. Online reservation, pre-examination, and triage should be implemented to redirect patients and avoid the overcrowding of patients in hospital. Inpatients are supposed to receive assessments to exclude COVID-19 before they are admitted to hospitals and visiting rules should be strict to avoid cross infection in hospitals.

24.2.2 *Community comprehensive preventive measures*

(1) One important measure to prevent COVID-19 is wearing masks meant for different levels of risk prevention. Choosing masks of

high-level prevention is unnecessary and costly, which could lead to the shortfall of masks for those in real need. Ordinary people are advised to wear disposable medical masks. People working in crowded areas, taking on certain jobs (such as policemen, security guards, and couriers), in home quarantine, and those who live with them, are advised to wear surgical masks or N95/K95 particulate masks, or masks of higher-level prevention of particulate matters. It is not suggested to use paper masks, activated carbon mask as well as cotton and gauze or sponge masks.

(2) Individuals are advised to keep good personal hygiene by washing hands frequently with soap, water, or alcohol-based sanitizer. They should cover their mouth and nose when coughing and sneezing, toss used tissues in sealed garbage, followed by washing hands with alcohol-based sanitizer and clean water, and avoid using hands to touch eyes, noses, and mouths.

(3) Keeping at least one meter away from others is necessary, particularly those who have coughing, sneezing, or fever. One should make fewer trips outside and avoid gatherings.

(4) Closing toilet lid before flushing could reduce aerosol concentration.

(5) One should keep rooms clean and ventilated, furniture free from dust, and clothes, beddings, and quilts should be changed frequently.

(6) The air supply of central air-conditioning in public space should be kept clean and the air supply equipment should be disinfected when necessary. Doors and windows should be opened regularly to maintain good indoor ventilation.

(7) Disinfection of object surface should be taken seriously since coronavirus on dry surfaces such as stainless steel, plastic, or cloth can survive more than one day.

According to *Diagnosis and Treatment Protocol for Novel Coronavirus Pneumonia* (*6th Trial Edition*), the virus is sensitive to ultraviolet light and heat, and it can be inactivated at 56°C for 30 minutes. Lipid solvents, such as ethyl ether, 75% ethanol, chlorine disinfectant, peracetic acid and chloroform can also effectively inactivate the virus, but chlorahexidine is an exception.

Research shows that coronavirus (both in suspension and dried on surfaces) is very susceptible to 70% ethanol, with reduction of viability by greater than 3 log within seconds. Thus, skin could be cleansed by or dipped in 75% ethanol for disinfection. However, ethanol should be kept away from fire sources and combustible materials since it is inflammable. It cannot be sprayed, splashed, or used for large-area disinfection, or increased concentration of ethanol in the air could start a fire.

For home disinfection, 75% ethanol or other chlorine disinfectants could be used to cleanse the object surface. When using chlorine disinfectants, one should pay attention to its preparation and dilution rate. In particular, one should avoid using chlorine disinfectants with other disinfectants to avoid producing large amount of poisonous gas. Heat-resistant products could be boiled for 15 minutes to get disinfected.

(8) Priorities should be given to the prevention and control of cluster outbreaks. Common gathering places include families, medical institutions, schools, shops, and hotels where there are usually clusters of people. Efforts should be made to raise the awareness of the severity of outbreak in clusters and mobilize the whole society to ban mass gatherings and close public areas.

Diamond Princess, a luxury cruise ship, carried 3,711 passengers and became the place with the most confirmed cases outside China during the early stage of the outbreak. With independent cabins floating on the sea, the ship seemed ideal for isolation. However, the number of confirmed cases went up quickly during isolation and working staff in charge of quarantine and transportation were also infected by the virus. According to available materials, its isolation measures did not meet the requirement of control and prevention at all. Its inner space was not compartmentalized in a right way. Possible infection areas were not separated from non-infection areas; passengers were allowed to move without restrictions; goods and products were passed from one area to another without restrictions; crew members were not in self-isolation, and they ate and drank together. It remains unclear whether cabins were completely isolated from each other despite seemingly independent, and whether its air supply system and the sewage system were up to standards. Diamond Princess is an unsuccessful model that shows simple isolation cannot stop the epidemic from spreading. Without effective measures to cut off its transmission channel, the whole ship became a hotbed of virus transmission.

24.2.3 *Protection of susceptible population*

SARS-CoV-2 is a new virus and the population is susceptible to it. Generally speaking, the main measure to protect susceptible population is through the use of vaccinations and drugs for prevention. Progress on vaccination development can be referred to in Chapter 3 of this book. To date, no clinical trials exist that prove certain drugs are effective in prevention. Healthy living habits, sufficient sleep, and a good state of mind are essential. Avoid feeling too nervous or stressed. Appropriate amount of physical activities after getting enough rest will also help to boost health and immunity.

Chapter 25
Prevention and Control
of Nosocomial Infection

During the COVID-19 epidemic, a large number of confirmed or suspected patients gathered in designated isolation hospitals; at the same time, patients with fever or respiratory symptoms have been constantly pouring into emergency and fever clinics. There is every possibility that these patients are the source of infection of the virus, thus exacerbating the spread of the epidemic. As frontline healthcare workers are the main force in fighting the epidemic, it is particularly important to block the spread of the virus in hospitals to protect medical staff and other personnel. China's National Health Commission statistics show that 1,716 medical personnel were diagnosed with COVID-19 nationwide as of 24:00 Feb 11, 2020, accounting for 3.8% of the total number of confirmed cases, with five dead. Hubei province reported 1,502 medical staff were confirmed having the infection, accounting for 87.5% of the national medical staff confirmed cases. Not only medical staff, but all personnel in the hospital are at risk of being infected by the virus during the outbreak. For example, Fuxing Hospital, Capital Medical University (Fuxing Hospital) encountered local viral transmission within departments caused by staff who had contact with externally infected people and became confirmed cases. As of February 19, 2020, Fuxing Hospital confirmed 34 cases and detected two nucleic acid positive cases. Among them were eight medical staff, 19 patients and their families, and nine nurses and cleaning staff.

In order to minimize the risk of infection of medical professionals, this chapter presents recommendations on infection prevention and control for professionals who may be exposed to patients and/or infectious sources (including patient's excreta, secretions, blood, and contaminated medical equipment, environmental surface, air, etc.).

25.1 Principles of Personal Protective Equipment Selection

Personal protective equipment (PPE) refers to tools used to protect medical personnel from exposure to infectious agents. According to *Guidelines for the Scope of Use of Common Medical Protective Equipment in the Prevention and Control of Pneumonia Infected by Novel Coronavirus (Trial)* issued by China's National Health Commission, this chapter will introduce PPE and the principles of selection related to this epidemic for proper selection in practical application.

25.1.1 *Goggles*

Goggles shall be used in areas such as observation wards (rooms), airborne infection isolation rooms (AIIRs), as well as during medical procedures where blood, body fluids, and secretions may splash, including collecting respiratory specimens, tracheal intubation, tracheotomy, non-invasive ventilation, and sputum suction. It is prohibited to leave the above areas wearing goggles. If the goggles are reusable, they shall be reused after disinfection, and special attention should be paid to the complete removal of residual disinfectants (such as chlorine-containing disinfectants) after disinfection so as not to cause adverse reactions to the eyes of medical staff. In principle, goggles should not be used in other areas, or for diagnosis and treatment in other areas.

25.1.2 *Masks/protective face shields*

Masks/protective face shields are used when blood, body fluids, and secretions may splatter during medical procedures. Reusable ones shall be disinfected before being reused; disposable ones must not be reused. There is no need to use goggles and masks/protective face shields at the same time. It is forbidden to leave the area wearing masks/protective face shields.

25.1.3 *Surgical masks*

Surgical masks shall be worn correctly to avoid failure in achieving protective effects. See instructions on proper wearing and removing of surgical masks below. Masks should be replaced as soon as they are contaminated or become wet.

25.1.4 *Medical protective masks*

Medical protective masks are in principle used in areas such as observation wards (rooms), AIIRs, and for operations that may generate aerosols, including collecting respiratory specimens, tracheal intubation, tracheostomy, noninvasive ventilation, and sputum suction. In principle, they should not be used in other areas, or for medical procedures in other areas. They should be worn correctly to avoid failure in achieving protective effects or contamination. See how to put on and take off masks correctly below. They are generally replaced once every 4 hours, and should be replaced as soon as they are contaminated or become wet.

25.1.5 *Latex examination gloves*

Latex examination gloves are used in areas such as pre-examination and triage, fever clinics, observation wards (rooms), and AIIRs. Gloves should be put on and taken off properly, and they should be used only once and changed promptly. It is forbidden to leave the clinic area with gloves. Wearing gloves cannot substitute for hand hygiene.

25.1.6 *Alcohol-containing hand sanitizer*

Alcohol-containing hand sanitizer should be used when there are no obvious contaminants on the hands of medical staff during their operations of diagnosis and treatment, and should be used throughout the hospital. Areas of pre-examination and triage, fever clinics, observation wards (rooms), and AIIRs must be equipped with alcohol-containing hand sanitizers.

25.1.7 *Surgical gowns*

Common isolation gowns are used in pre-examination triage and fever outpatient areas, while disposable impermeable isolation gowns are used in observation wards (rooms) and AIIRs. Isolation gowns may be used in other departments or areas based on whether there is contact with patients. Disposable isolation gowns must not be reused. For reusable isolation gowns, disinfect them according to regulations before reuse. It is prohibited to leave the above areas wearing surgical gowns.

25.1.8 *Protective gown coveralls*

Protective gown coveralls are used in observation wards (rooms) and AIIRs for COVID-19 patients. In principle, protective gown coveralls should not be used in other areas, or for diagnoses and treatments in other areas. They must not be reused, and it is forbidden to leave the above areas while wearing them. Protective gown coveralls can be used continuously when contacting multiple confirmed patients; they should be replaced when contacting different suspected cases. Protective gown coveralls should be replaced promptly if they are contaminated by the blood and body fluids of patients. They must be put on and taken off correctly. See below for the proper way of donning and removing them.

Other personnel, such as sanitation workers and security, should use protective equipment according to protection requirements of the relevant area, and wear and remove protective gown coveralls correctly.

25.2 Protection Levels

According to different protection requirements, the protection levels are divided as follows.

25.2.1 *Level I protection*

Work clothes, disposable medical caps, surgical gowns, medical surgical masks, and if necessary, disposable gloves.

25.2.2 *Level II protection*

Medical protective masks, disposable medical caps, impermeable disposable isolation gowns or protective gown coveralls, gloves, shoe covers, and if necessary, goggles or protective face shields.

25.2.3 *Level III protection*

Medical protective masks, disposable medical caps, protective gown coveralls, gloves, shoe covers, goggles or protective face shields, and if necessary, powered air-purifying respirators (PAPRs).

25.3 Self-Protection Requirements for Medical Personnel in Different Areas

25.3.1 *Hospital entrance and outpatient department*

Medical personnel who maintain order and take body temperature at hospital entrance shall wear medical surgical masks; medical personnel inquiring about epidemiological information shall wear goggles, disposable medical caps, medical protective masks, isolation gowns, and gloves. Outpatient medical staff, other than fever clinics, shall wear medical surgical masks.

25.3.2 *Emergency*

Staff in the pre-examination triage and emergency rescue area should wear disposable medical caps, goggles, medical protective masks, surgical gowns, and gloves.

25.3.3 *Fever clinics and observation wards*

Medical personnel in fever clinics should wear isolation gowns, disposable medical caps, gloves, medical protective masks, goggles or face shields, and shoe covers during daily medical activities. Medical personnel in observation wards should wear protective gown coveralls, disposable medical caps, gloves, medical protective masks, goggles or face shields, and shoe covers during daily medical activities.

When performing operations that may generate aerosols or splashes, such as collecting respiratory specimens, tracheal intubations, bronchoscopy, and airway sputum suctions, medical personnel should wear protective gown coveralls, disposable medical caps, gloves, and powered air-purifying respirators. Staff accompanying patients to fever clinics should wear medical surgical masks, disposable medical caps, isolation gowns, and if necessary, goggles.

25.3.4 *Other areas of medical institutions*

Medical staff in other wards should wear medical surgical masks and goggles or face shields if necessary. Staff from auxiliary medical departments, such as pathology and radiology, should wear medical surgical masks and may choose medical protective masks in some high-risk situations. In places with no close contact with patients such as functional departments and logistics departments, ordinary medical masks shall be adequate. However, if a suspected COVID-19 case occurs in the above departments, self-protection of personnel should be performed according to the standards of fever clinics and observation wards. If resources are limited, the medical protective masks can be replaced with particulate respirators (such as N95, KN95, and FFP2) for medical personnel in non-fever clinics and non-isolation areas.

25.4 Donning and Removing Procedures of Personal Protective Equipment

25.4.1 *Surgical masks*

Perform hand hygiene before putting on a surgical mask. The deep colored side of the mask faces outward, with the metallic strip uppermost. Two pairs of strings are tied behind the head in parallel, with one pair tied behind the neck and the other on ears. Use both hands to squeeze the metallic strips on the nose, pull out the folds of the mask with both hands to ensure that the mask can fit snugly over the face, and cover the nose and chin completely (Figure 25-1).

When removing the mask, pull only the straps to avoid touching both sides of the mask. Try to close eyes and hold breath, and dispose

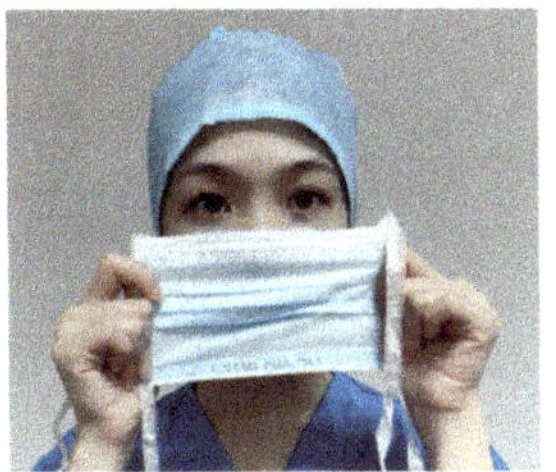

(1) Perform hand hygiene before wearing the mask, with the deep colored side facing outward and the metallic nose clip uppermost.

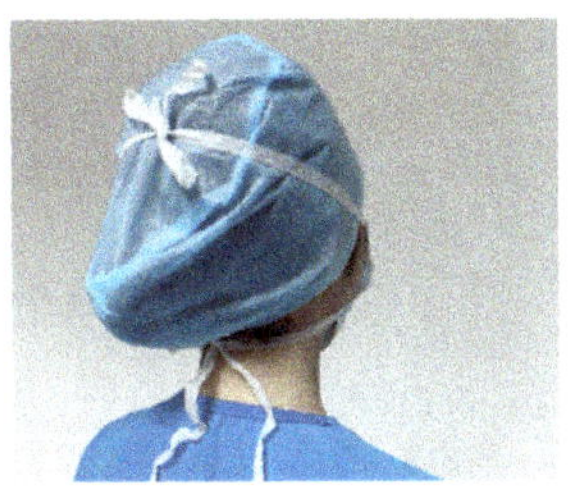

(2) Tie the straps behind the head and neck respectively.

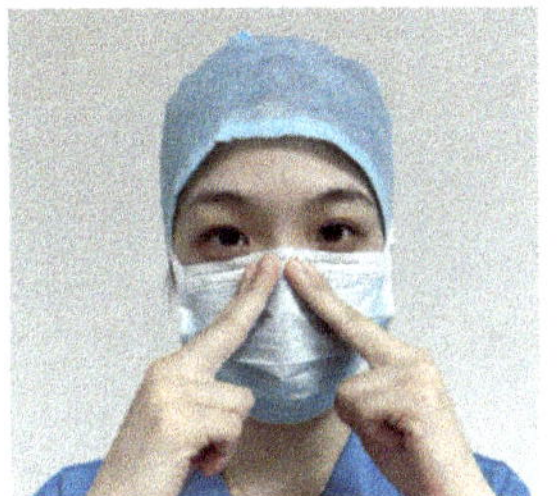

(3) Press the metallic nose clip inward until it is pressed into the shape of a nose bridge.

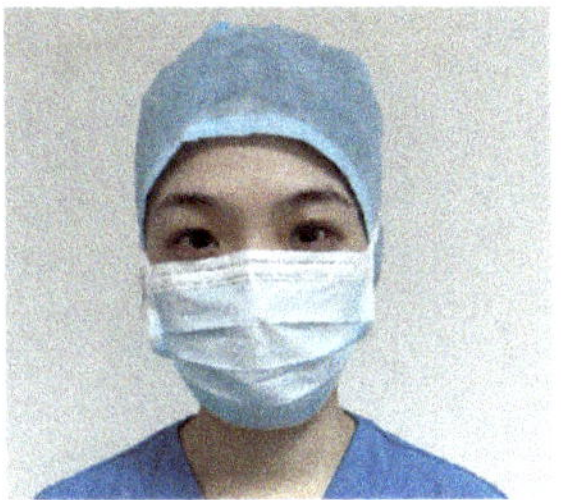

(4) After completion, the mask must cover the nose to chin.

Figure 25-1.   Wearing a disposable medical mask

of the mask into a biohazard trash can. Do not wear one mask for more than four hours.

25.4.2 *Protective masks*

Perform hand hygiene before wearing the mask. Hold the mask with one hand and cup it on the face. Place the lower strap behind the neck, then the upper strap on the ears, with the two straps parallel behind the head. Press the nose clip with both hands to make the mask fit snugly over the face. Press the front of the mask with both hands to perform a tightness test: when exhaling deeply, a positive pressure indicates no air leakage; when inhaling deeply, the mask close against face indicates no air leakage. Adjust the mask position or tighten the straps if there is air leakage (Figure 25-2).

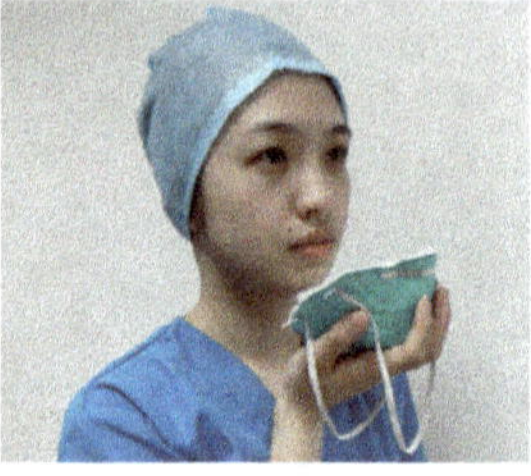

(1) Perform hand hygiene before wearing
the mask, hold it with hand in the shape
of a cup, with the straps sagging naturally.

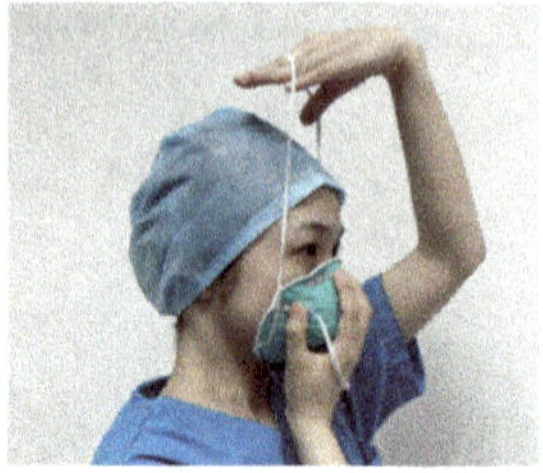

(2) Put the mask in a proper position with the
metal nose clip upward. Loop the lower strap
over the head and place under the ears.

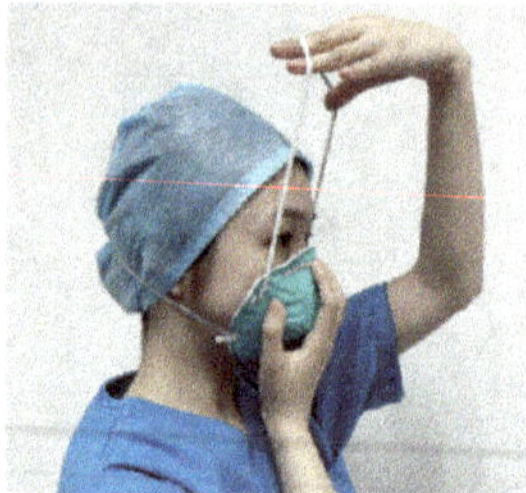

(3) Fix the upper strap at a higher position
at the back of the head.

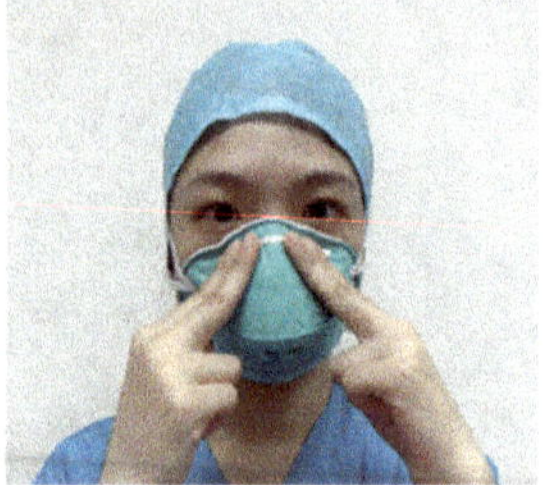

(4) Adjust the shape of nose clip with
fingers of both hands.

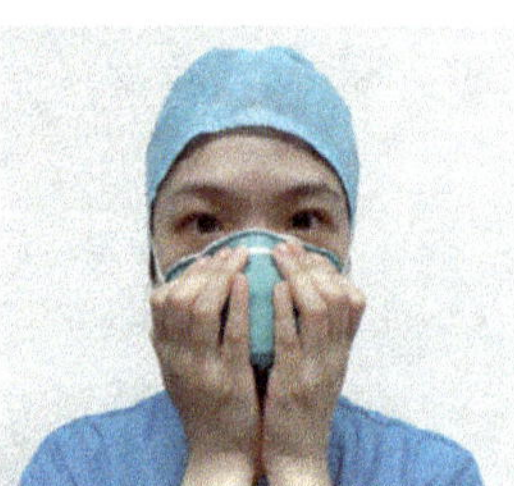

(5) Check tightness: cover the mask completely
with both hands and exhale quickly.
Adjust the nose clip if there is leakage near it.
Adjust the position of the straps if there is
leakage around the mask.

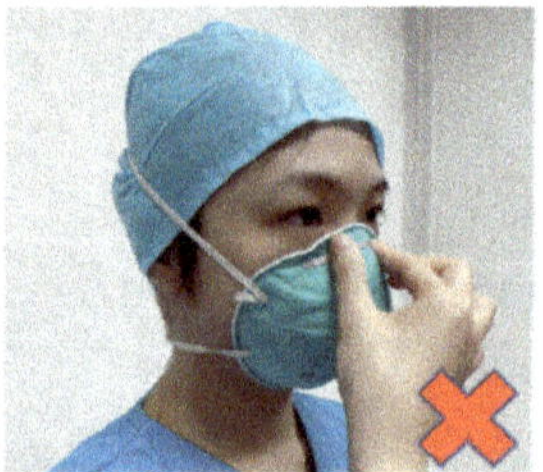

Note: Do not adjust the nose clip
with one hand,
which may cause air
leakage and affect the use of masks.

Figure 25-2.   Wearing a medical protective mask

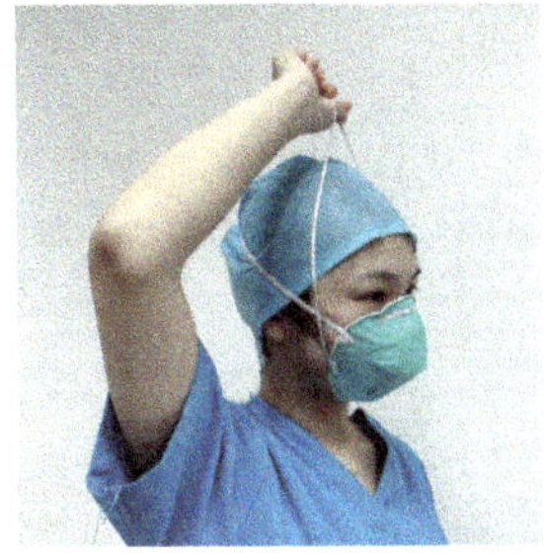

(1) When removing the mask,
pull the lower strap over the top of head
and release it.

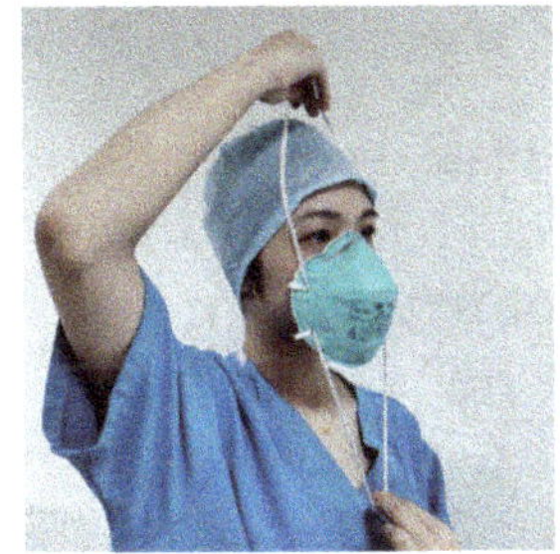

(2) Pull the upper strap over the top of
the head, take the strap to remove the mask
from the lower front, and pull the lower strap
with the other hand to avoid the mask from
springing up. Do not touch the front of the mask.

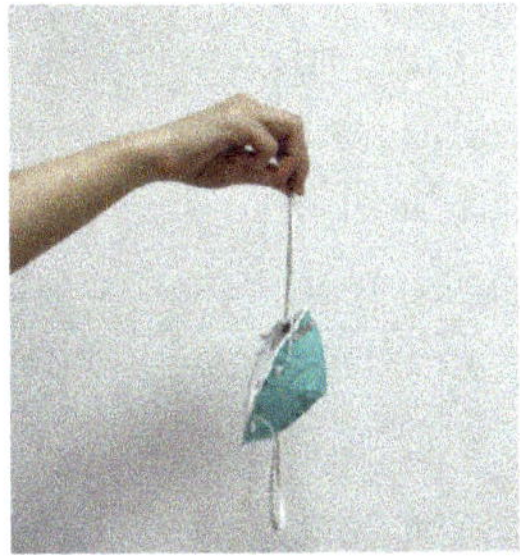

(3) When removing the mask, pull only the straps to avoid
touching both sides of the mask. Try to close eyes and hold breath,
and throw the mask into a biohazard trash can.

Figure 25-3.   Removing a mask

When taking off the mask, pull the lower strap over the top of the head and loosen it. Then pull the upper strap over the top of the head, and use the strap to remove the mask from the lower front without touching the front of the mask. When removing the mask, pull only the straps to avoid touching both sides of the mask. Close eyes and hold breath if possible, then perform hand hygiene immediately after disposing the mask into a biohazard trash can (Figure 25-3). Do not wear one mask for more than four hours.

25.4.3 *Disposable surgical gowns*

Perform hand hygiene before removing isolation gown. Untie the straps behind surgical gown. Withdraw hands from sleeves, and be careful not to touch the outside of surgical gown. Remove the surgical gown from the inside and dispose of it into a biohazard trash can. Perform hand hygiene at the end.

25.4.4 *Protective gown coveralls*

When removing protective gown coveralls, open the seal and zipper first, and then perform hand hygiene and take off the outer gloves. Remove the protective cap from the inside, and then take off the sleeves. Be careful not to touch the outside of the protective gown coveralls with hands. Grasp the inner side with both hands, gently roll it outward to the ankles, and remove the protective gown coveralls together with shoe covers (if any). Dispose of it into a biohazard trash can. Perform hand hygiene (Figure 25-4) at the end.

25.4.5 *Goggles/protective face shields*

Adjust to a comfortable state after wearing goggles/protective face shields, and perform hand hygiene before removing them. Grasp the ear circumference of the goggles or the end of the head circumference of the protective face shields to remove the goggles.

Do not touch the front of goggles/protective face shields with hands. Place the reusable ones in a container with a lid for centralized cleaning and disinfection, and throw the non-reusable ones directly into a biohazard trash can. Perform hand hygiene at the end.

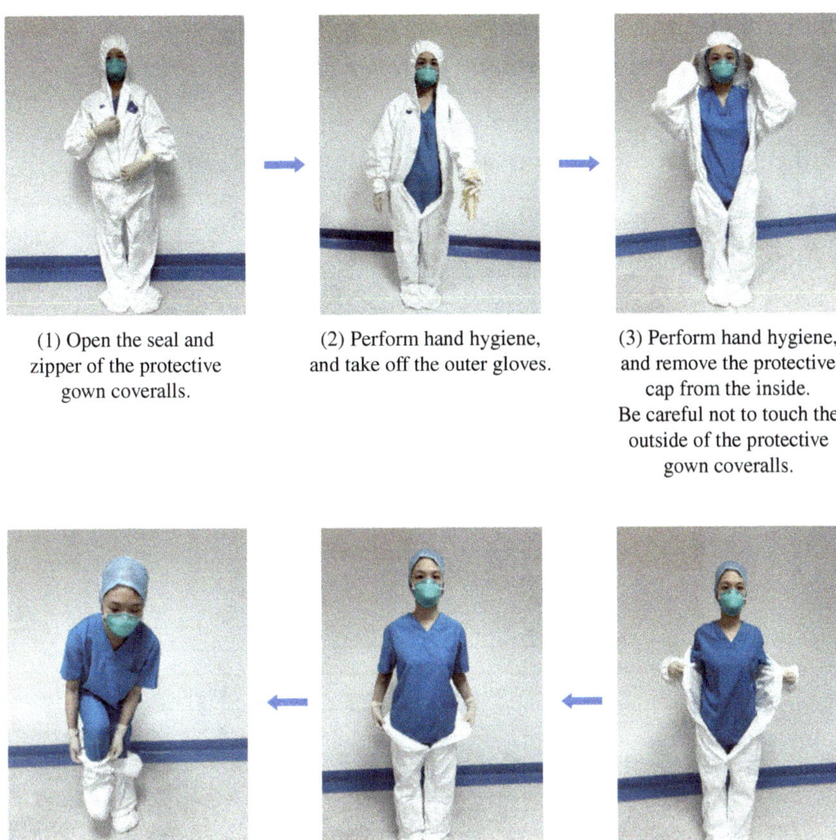

(1) Open the seal and zipper of the protective gown coveralls.

(2) Perform hand hygiene, and take off the outer gloves.

(3) Perform hand hygiene, and remove the protective cap from the inside. Be careful not to touch the outside of the protective gown coveralls.

(4) Grasp the inner side with both hands, take off the sleeves, gently roll it outward to the ankles, and take it off together with shoe covers (if any). Throw it into a biohazard trash can.

Figure 25-4. Removing a protective gown coveralls

25.4.6 *The donning and removing process of personal protective equipment in fever clinics and AIIRs*

(1) Enter the contaminated zone: see Figure 25-5.
(2) Leave the contaminated zone: see Figures 25-6 and 25-7.

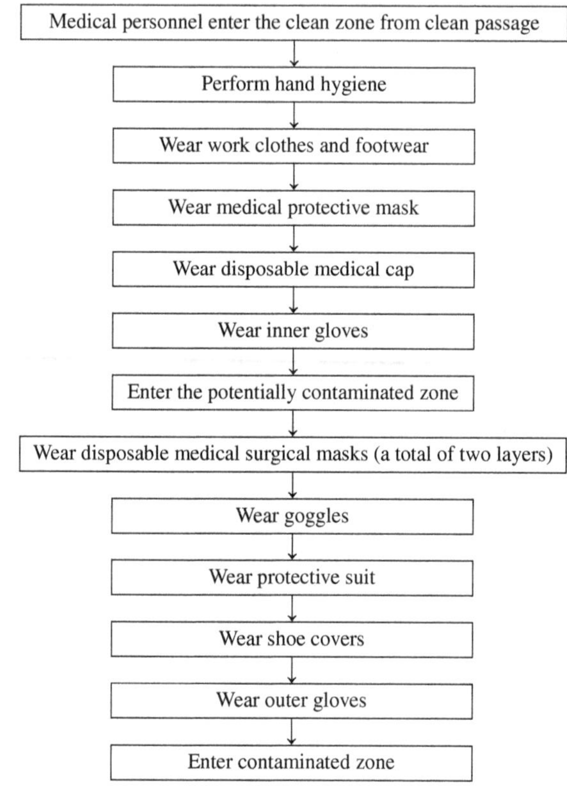

Figure 25-5.   Flow chart of medical staff entering contaminated zones

Note: If high-risk operations that may generate aerosol are involved, a powered, air-purifying respirator (PAPR) is required (level III protection).

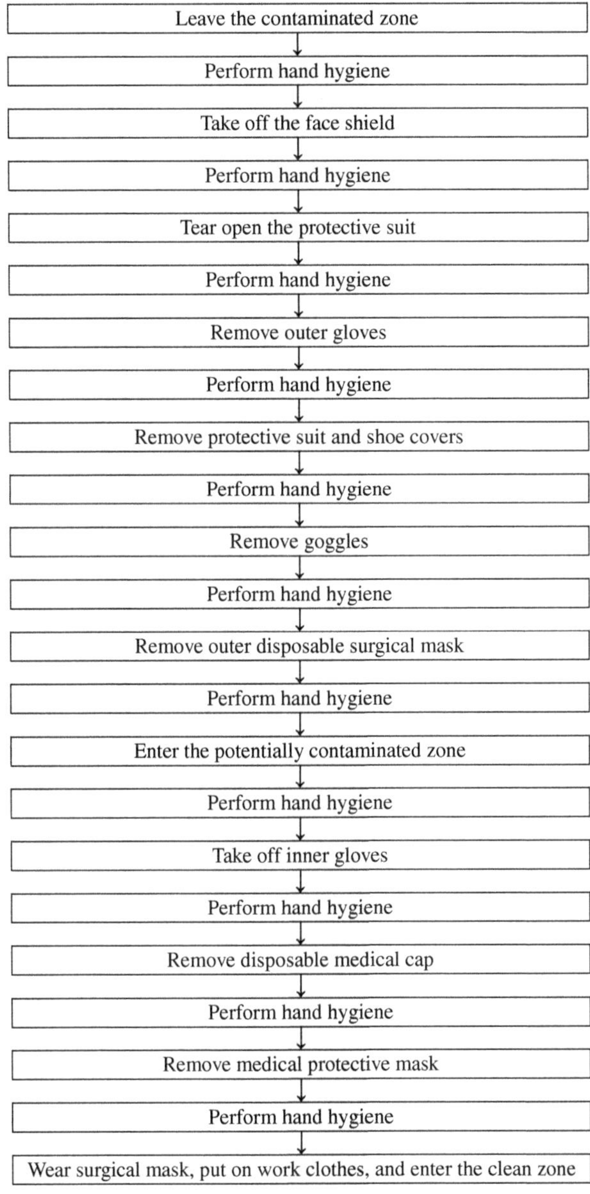

Figure 25-6.   Flow chart of medical staff leaving the contaminated zone

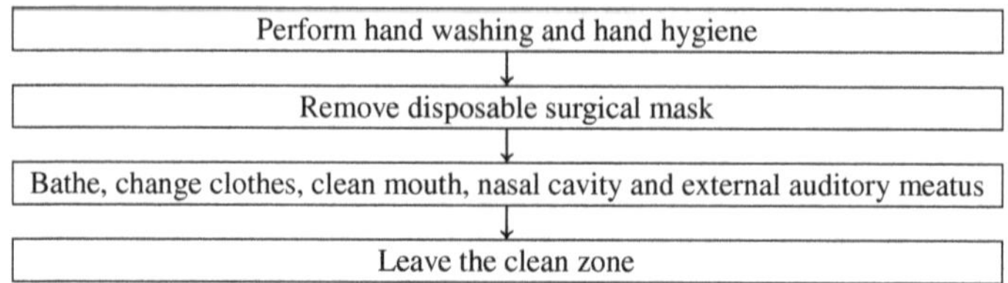

Figure 25-7.　Flow chart of medical staff leaving the clean zone before off-duty

25.4.7 *Protection procedures during transfer of confirmed patients*

(1) The process of wearing protective items: see Figure 25-8.

(2) The process of removing protective items: see Figure 25-9.

(3) Transfer process: carry patients with a negative pressure ambulance and instruct them to wear surgical masks. Transfer patients to designated isolation medical institutions. After transferring, staff return to the original location in the special transfer ambulance. Clean the special ambulance, and open windows for ventilation. Spray 1-3% hydrogen peroxide, 0.5% peroxyacetic acid, or disinfectant solution containing 1000 mg/L of available chlorine on the vehicle interior and exterior surfaces and the object surfaces in the vehicle for 30 minutes until wet. Only after disinfection the next patient can be transferred.

It should be pointed out that "behavior barrier" is more important than "physical barrier". Medical personnel should receive strict training on prevention and control of nosocomial infections, making sure that basic concepts such as "contamination", "cleaning", and "isolation" are well understood. Especially at present, many medical institutions are still restrained to limited conditions (such as the division of "clean zone, potentially contaminated zone, contaminated zone and clean passage, contaminated passage"). Therefore, medical personnel's regulating their own behaviors is even more important under this circumstance.

In addition, the key to the proper use of protective equipment is not to blindly upgrade protection level or put on more protective equipment than needed, but to focus on selecting and using personal

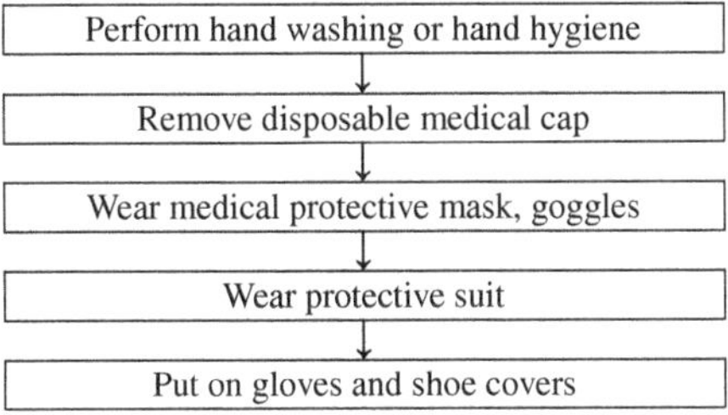

Figure 25-8. Flow chart of wearing protective equipment for confirmed patients

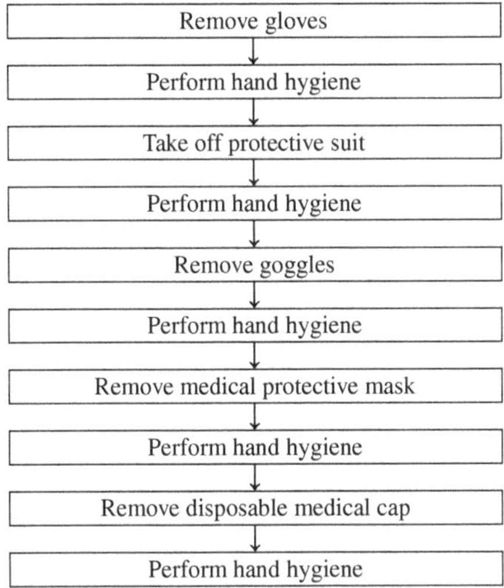

Figure 25-9. Flow chart of removing protective equipment for confirmed patients

protective equipment correctly. Otherwise, it would only lead to the wastage of medical resources and decreased protective effect.

25.5 Cleaning and Disinfection Process of Air, Environment and Surface

25.5.1 *Air disinfection*

Disinfection staff shall, according to the protection requirements of each area mentioned above, wear personal protective equipment correctly. Choose air disinfection measures according to the region's setup and actual situation. For non-negative pressure wards, perform natural ventilation or mechanical ventilation, ultraviolet radiation, and use air sterilizer 2 to 3 times a day, ≥ 30 minutes each time. In negative pressure areas, according to Requirements of Environmental Control for Hospital Negative Pressure Isolation Ward (GB/T 35428-2017), make sure that airflow goes from clean zones → potentially contaminated zones → contaminated zones, and maintain a certain negative pressure difference between areas. The pressure difference between adjacent areas should ≥5Pa; the order of negative pressure from high to low is AIIR toilets (–15Pa) → AIIRs (–10Pa) → buffer rooms (–5Pa) → potentially contaminated zone corridors (–5Pa). Maintain positive air pressure in clean zones (0Pa), relative to outdoor atmospheric pressure. Keep the frequency of ventilation in negative pressure AIIRs' contaminated zones and potentially contaminated zones at 10–15 times/hour. After discharge of COVID-19 patients, replace air outlet filters of the negative pressure ward timely, and clean the inner surfaces of the air outlet with disinfectants. Record air disinfection history afterwards.

25.5.2 *Air conditioning management*

Turn down or completely close return air valves, open all the new air valves, and turn on air exhausting systems if medical institutions use air-conditioning systems during the epidemic; clean and disinfect filter screens, filters, supply-air outlets, and return-air inlets once a week, using disinfectant containing 250–500 mg/L of active chlorine (bromine) or chlorine dioxide to spray, immerse or wipe for 10–30 minutes.

Once a suspected or confirmed case occurs in a building, air-conditioning ventilation systems should be shut down immediately, and restarted only after effective cleaning and disinfection. During air fumigating disinfection of patients' room, stand-alone air conditioners should be kept running while the direct air conditioner should be turned off. After air disinfection, doors and windows should be opened, and air-conditioning systems should be turned on to maximum for air extraction for a period of time. Filter screens and filters should be disinfected before being replaced. Disinfectant solution containing 2000 mg/L active chlorine is recommended. Spray items with the solution for 30 minutes until wet. Old filter screens and filters should be removed, disinfected, and burned. All air supply equipment and pipes should be disinfected with 1000–2000 mg/L active chlorine (bromine)-containing solution for 30 minutes. Fumigate with peracetic acid (1 g/m³) or spray with 0.5% peracetic acid solution, which can be used for disinfecting air handling units. The units should be sealed for 60 minutes and then ventilated. The air-conditioning condensate should be collected in a sealed container, and then treated as medical sewage, by adding chlorine (bromine) disinfectant, with 200 mg/L of active chlorine (bromine). Drain the condensate after mixing them for 1 hour. For continuous collection, add disinfection solution containing 500 mg/L active chlorine (bromine) to collection container in advance. Cover the container to avoid aerosols. For medical institutions that shut down air-conditioning systems during the epidemic, cleaning and disinfection, as well as replacement of certain units should be carried out by certified professional institutions after the epidemic.

25.5.3 *Cleaning and disinfection of goggles, face shields, and powered air-purifying respirators (PAPRs)*

After use, disinfect goggles thoroughly with hydrogen peroxide wipes and dry them. For face shields, remove disposable plastic sheets and dispose of them into biohazard fabric bag. Immerse the reusable parts with 2000 mg/L active chlorine-containing disinfectant for 30 minutes, and then rinse and dry them thoroughly. Hydrogen peroxide wipes are also suitable.

Powered air-purifying respirators (PAPRs) can be disinfected with hydrogen peroxide wipes if not contaminated by blood or other body fluids. If contaminated, rinse with running water first, and then disinfect. Remove and dispose of the filter box into a biohazard fabric bag if it is contaminated with blood or other body fluids. Rinse the rest of the parts with running water, and then disinfect with hydrogen peroxide wipes.

25.5.4 *Cleaning and disinfection of thermometers*

For thermometers used in pre-examination triage, fever clinics, AIIRs, wipe the surface with 75% ethanol, immerse them in a disinfectant containing 1000 mg/L of active chlorine for 30 minutes, rinse the residual disinfectant with clean water, and dry them with gauze for use. For thermometers used by non-COVID-19 patients, wipe the surface with 75% ethanol, then soak with 75% ethanol or disinfectant containing 500 mg/L of active chlorine for 30 minutes. Rinse off the residual disinfectant with clean water, and then dry with gauze.

25.5.5 *Cleaning and disinfection of medical devices such as laryngoscope, bronchoscope, and negative pressure suction bottle*

Regular cleaning and disinfection process should be carried out as usual. Except for parts that require cleansing from professionals, all the external surfaces, reusable parts, and cleaning tanks should be wiped or immersed for 30 minutes using a disinfectant solution containing 1000 mg/L active chlorine, hydrogen peroxide, ethanol, etc. Used disposable parts shall be treated as COVID-19 medical waste.

Note that level III protection should be taken when cleaning negative pressure suction bottles. It should be opened in the biohazard waste room, then added disinfectant containing 2000 mg/L active chlorine. Mix the disinfectant and leave the bottles for 2 hours before dumping the content into hospital sewage pipes. Bottles used by suspected or confirmed COVID-19 patients should be first immersed completely in a 2000 mg/L active chlorine-containing disinfectant for 30 minutes. Then rinse the suction bottles, accessories, and pipes under running water to remove obvious contaminants. Clean every part using a dedicated brush and running water, and immerse them completely in a covered container with 1000 mg/L active chlorine-containing disinfectant for 30 minutes. Staff wearing long-sleeved thick rubber gloves should remove residual disinfectant thoroughly with running water. Dry the surface of the bottle and accessories, as well as the inside of the pipelines. Place them in clean sealed plastic bags after assembling.

25.5.6 *Cleaning and disinfection of clinic areas for suspected or confirmed cases*

Areas with suspected or confirmed cases should be ventilated at least 2–3 times a day, ≥30 minutes each time. Use mechanical ventilation if necessary. In the absence of people, ultraviolet or hydrogen peroxide may be employed to disinfect the air and surfaces of objects. Alternatively, use 1–3% hydrogen peroxide solution, disinfection solution with 1000 mg/L active chlorine wipes to clean the surfaces. Boil reusable medical fabrics for 10 minutes, or soak with a disinfectant containing 1000 mg/L active chlorine for 30 minutes before performing standard cleaning and disinfection. The same applies for tableware. For floor contaminated with blood or body fluids, cover with towels with disinfectant for at least one hour before cleaning and disinfecting. All wastes should be put in double-layer biohazard bags and sent to solid waste centers for incineration as infectious waste.

25.5.7 *Cleaning and disinfection of reusable sanitary products*

Sanitary products should not be used across rooms in the fever clinic and AIIRs. Used disinfectant wipes should be treated as infectious waste. Place the reusable sanitary items in a particular container with 2000 mg/L active chlorine (bromide)-containing disinfectant for 30 minutes. After rinsing and draining, put them into double-layer biohazard fabric bags, tighten, and label the bags. They should be sent to cleaning company for mechanical cleaning and thermal drying for future use.

25.5.8 *Cleaning and disinfection of medical fabrics*

Fabrics used by patients and medical staff in fever clinics and AIIRs should be gathered into orange-red collection bags with "infectious fabrics" logo by the patient's bed. Spray and disinfect the bag with 1000 mg/L active chlorine-containing solution before sealing. Do not exceed 2/3 of the loading capacity. Keep it sealed until washing.

25.5.9 *Cleaning and disinfection of bed unit in AIIRs after patients' discharge*

Cleaners should take level II protection. Disinfect air using aerosol spray of 0.5% peroxyacetic acid, 1–3% hydrogen peroxide or 500 mg/L chlorine dioxide, with 20 ml/m³ for 1 hour. Open windows or use mechanical ventilation for 30 minutes. Pack fabrics as described above. Disinfect surfaces as described above, then clean them with water (cleaning sequence: from top to bottom, from inside to outside, from mild pollution to serious pollution. Remove small amounts of contaminants carefully using disposable absorbent materials. For large amounts of contaminants, cover them completely with disposable absorbent materials, and then spray disinfectant solution with 5000–10000 mg/L of active chlorine till wet. After 30 minutes, transfer the contaminants carefully to medical waste container. Avoid contact with contaminants. Disinfect contaminated surfaces with disinfectant containing 2000 mg/L of active chlorine. In the observation room, if the patient is ruled out of having COVID-19, the final cleaning and disinfection can be handled as usual. If the patient is diagnosed with the disease, follow the procedures described above.

25.5.10 *Infected operating room*

After surgery for a COVID-19 patient is finished, perform air disinfection first. For negative pressure operating rooms, shut down the laminar flow and air supply, and disinfect the air using peracetic acid/hydrogen peroxide spray for 1–2 hours. Turn on negative pressure laminar flows and ventilation for 30 minutes. Inform personnel in charge to replace high-efficiency filters in negative pressure operating rooms promptly. For routine infection operation rooms, disinfect the air using peracetic acid/hydrogen peroxide spray for 1–2 hours. After air disinfection, cleaning staff should take level II protection. Clean the floor and surfaces of equipment and devices using a disinfectant with 1000 mg/L active chlorine, and leave for 30 minutes before wiping with clean water. For surfaces contaminated by patients' blood, body fluids, etc., wipe with 5000 mg/L chlorine disinfectant. Pre-treat reusable medical devices with a disinfectant containing

1000 mg/L active chlorine, before sealing in double-layer yellow fabric bags. Put them in transfer boxes labeled "COVID-19" and transport to supply rooms by dedicated staff. Disposable medical supplies are treated as medical waste.

25.5.11 *Cleaning and disinfection of elevators*

COVID-19 patients and other people should not use the same elevator, and elevators should be clearly marked. For normal elevators, clean and disinfect the walls, buttons, and floor for more than 30 minutes with a disinfectant solution containing 500 mg/L active chlorine, and then wipe with clean water. Dedicated elevators for COVID-19 patients should have warning signs. Cleaning staff should take level I protection. Clean and disinfect elevator walls, keys, and floor with disinfectant containing 1000 mg/L active chlorine for more than 30 minutes, then wipe with clean water. Disposable PPE should be handled properly as described before.

25.5.12 *Precautions for cleaning and disinfection*

SARS-CoV-2 is a lipophilic virus and is sensitive to a variety of disinfectants including 75% ethanol, peroxide, and chlorine-containing disinfectants. Select the type and effective concentration of disinfectant correctly according to previous recommendations. As for the most commonly used chlorine-containing disinfectant for surface disinfection, the concentration of active chlorine should be increased accordingly as the potential viral loads increase. It is not necessary to make the concentration higher than needed, because disinfectants can cause adverse reactions. Therefore, select the appropriate concentration according to the situation. On the other hand, sufficient duration of disinfection should be ensured, not less than 30 minutes.

During the disinfection process, note the following possible issues.

Cleaning personnel should be careful about personal protection when performing disinfection, avoiding contact of disinfectants with the skin, mucous membranes, and respiratory tract. At the same time, ensure containers filled with disinfectant are sealed to minimize volatilization of the disinfectant and generation of aerosols. For reusable personal protective equipment such as goggles and protective face shields, cleaning personnel should make sure the residual disinfectant solution is completely removed to avoid irritation and adverse reactions to the users' conjunctiva and skin during the next use.

When selecting a disinfectant, pay attention to the expiration date of the disinfectant and avoid using an invalid disinfectant. Generally, the validity period of sealed volatile alcohol products after opening is no more than 30 days, and that of non-volatile products is no more than 60 days. The validity period of a chlorine-containing disinfectant is generally no more than 24 hours, and its chlorine concentration can be measured with chlorine test paper.

The combination of disinfectants may be contraindicated as some mixtures can result in reduced effectiveness or even toxic substances. Common contraindicated combinations such as quaternary ammonium disinfectants (such as benzalkonium bromide bromo-geramine) are cationic surfactants. When mixed with anionic surfactants like soap, it will produce an antagonistic effect and reduce its disinfecting effect. Similarly, quaternary ammonium disinfectants cannot be used together with iodine or peroxides (such as potassium permanganate and hydrogen peroxide). Chloride-containing disinfectants are alkaline, while most of the toilet detergents are strongly acidic. When mixed, the two will react violently and produce a large amount of toxic chlorine gas.

25.6 Management of Relevant Departments

25.6.1 *Outpatient and triage*

Staff should wear work clothes, goggles, isolation gowns, disposable medical caps, medical protective masks, and gloves. After investigation about epidemiological history and taking body temperature for suspected cases, they should personally accompany suspected patients to the fever clinics. Keep 1.5-meter distance. Perform routine cleaning and disinfection at the end of each shift for the triage table and surrounding environment.

25.6.2 *Fever clinics*

Fever clinics should keep a reasonable architectural layout and a clear distinction of clean and contaminated zones. Better ventilation is required and air-conditioning system should be independent. Equip the entrance and clinics with alcohol-containing hand sanitizer. Enough observation rooms should be provided. Isolate and report suspected cases promptly. It is recommended to divide clinic rooms into special rooms (specifically for patients with a high possibility of COVID-19) and general rooms (for fever patients with clear causes or patients with less possibility of COVID-19).

All patients should wear medical surgical masks. Medical institutions should provide masks for patients and their escorts and guide them to wear masks correctly. Make sure that the waiting zones are well ventilated and not crowded. Patients with relevant epidemiological history should wait in a separate area.

Medical personnel should carry out hand hygiene strictly as recommended. Choose appropriate personal protective equipment and follow standard procedures to don and remove personal protective equipment. Medical staff should fully understand the epidemiological and clinical features of COVID-19 patients. Perform patient screening according to clinical norms. Take immediate isolation measures for suspected or confirmed patients, and report to relevant department at once.

Clean and disinfect the air, surfaces, and floor daily. After discharging patients, perform final disinfection.

25.6.3 *Emergency room*

Isolation zones should be set aside where practical in emergency departments for local isolation and treatment of suspected or diagnosed patients. When entering emergency room, medical personnel should wear work clothes, disposable medical caps, medical protective masks, surgical gowns, goggles or face shields, and disposable latex examination gloves. When inquiring about the epidemiological history and related clinical symptoms, medical staff should measure the vital signs of the patients. Patients should wear surgical masks. For suspected cases, they should be immediately transferred to isolated single rooms or isolated zones. Dedicated passages should be set up to transfer them to observation wards. After transferring the suspected patients, perform standardized cleaning and disinfection of wards.

25.6.4 *Outpatient clinics*

Outpatient clinics include general outpatient clinics and specialty departments such as stomatology, endoscopy, and obstetrics and gynecology. Pre-examination should screen out suspected patients with epidemiological history, and they should be guided to fever clinics. Control the number of patients, and try to keep the distance between patients at more than 1.5 meters in waiting rooms. Patients coming to departments such as stomatology and endoscopic should be postponed if not urgent. Make sure that there are no more than one patient in a room. Medical personnel should wear work clothes, disposable medical caps, and medical surgical masks (wear medical protective masks, latex gloves, disposable impermeable isolation gowns, goggles or protective face shields in special departments such as stomatology and endoscopy). For suspected patients, guiding personnel should accompany them to fever clinics and then perform disinfection of the clinics as well as the surroundings. Suspected patients in obstetrics department should be directed to dedicated prenatal examination room and examined by staff with level II protection. The internal environment of departments of stomatology should be disinfected after use. Endoscopes in endoscopic clinics should be disinfected according to standard regulations.

25.6.5 *Predelivery and delivery of pregnant women with COVID-19*

Parturient women should wear medical surgical masks and be transported to isolated delivery rooms by special personnel to wait for delivery. Medical personnel should take level II protection, wear sterile surgical gowns and double-layer gloves for delivery. After newborns are delivered, observe the mothers for two hours, and transfer them to the AIIRs by special personnel if there is no abnormality. The placenta, medical waste, and medical devices should be treated according to relevant procedures. Cleaning staff should take level II protection to disinfect isolated delivery rooms. Medical personnel should take off protective equipment in accordance with specifications and requirements.

25.6.6 *Hemodialysis room*

Pay attention to the temperature monitoring and epidemiological history inquiry of hemodialysis patients. If there is no relevant information, patients should wear masks to enter the hemodialysis zone for normal hemodialysis. If there is relevant information, patients should wear masks and be accompanied by special personnel to the fever observation rooms. Staff should wear level II protection equipment and perform hemodialysis for patients. It is important to thoroughly disinfect the surface and internal piping of the hemodialysis machine after use.

25.6.7 *Operating room*

For COVID-19 patients who need surgery, negative pressure operating rooms should be prepared, and laminar flow should be closed in non-negative pressure operating rooms. Before entering operating rooms, all surgical personnel should wear medical protective masks, goggles, medical protective gowns, latex gloves, and if necessary, face shields or powered air-purifying respirators. Medical personnel on the operating table should implement hand hygiene, and wear goggles, protective gown coverall, full instep protective shoes with shoe covers, and face shields or air-powered purified ventilator if necessary. After entering the operating room, they should wear the first layer of sterile medical gloves and disposable sterile impermeable surgical gowns, and the second layer of sterile medical gloves. Note that the operating rooms should be marked with "Novel Coronavirus" to restrict access to unrelated personnel.

26.6.8 *General ward*

Apart from AIIRs, emergency AIIRs should also be set up in ordinary ward area for suspected or confirmed cases, and related work systems and procedures should be established. Adequate disinfection and protective equipment for coping with acute respiratory infectious diseases should also be prepared. If a suspected or confirmed patient is found in the ward (room), relevant contingency plans and work processes should be initiated. Prompt and effective isolation, treatment, and referral should be implemented in accordance with specifications. Suspected or confirmed patients should be diagnosed and cared for by dedicated personnel. Access to unrelated medical personnel should be restricted. In principle, visiting is not allowed and if possible, patients can be placed in AIIRs. For non-designated hospitals without conditions for treatment, patients should be transferred to designated hospitals with isolation and treatment capabilities in a timely manner. While waiting for a referral, patients should be isolated and treated with effective measures. After transferring patients, the environment that patients are exposed to should be disinfected in accordance with the "Technical Standard for Disinfection of Medical and Health Structures".

Before starting routine medical care, medical staff should measure the vital signs of patients already in hospitals and newly admitted patients. If patients have fever and/or respiratory symptoms or epidemiological history, medical staff should instruct them (including escort person) to correctly wear medical surgical masks, immediately transfer them to emergency isolation rooms, and implement single-room isolation; medical personnel should report to relevant departments, perform laboratory tests or radiological examinations, and comprehensively determine whether to exclude or diagnose suspected cases. If diagnosis is planned, the patient should be transferred to the AIIRs or designated hospital. Final disinfection of the related environment should be performed.

A reasonable visitation system should be established for inpatients: other personnel are not recommended to visit hospitalized patients to avoid cross infection. If the patient needs an escort, each patient should have one relatively fixed person in principle, and escorts cannot be changed at will. Observe the hospital visiting time. Only one person is allowed to visit at a time, and the visiting time shall not exceed one hour. Strictly screen the visitors, register their information, examine body temperature, and investigate epidemiology. In particular , pay special attention to visitors' fever, respiratory symptoms, epidemiological history, including whether they have travel or residence history within 14 days to/in Wuhan or other areas still having spread of local cases; whether they have been exposed within the past 14 days to patients with fever or respiratory symptoms, who are from Wuhan or other areas having spread of local cases; and whether they are epidemiologically associated with clustered onset or confirmed cases, mild cases, and asymptomatic cases. Anyone involved in one of the above is not allowed to enter the ward. Asymptomatic cases with history of epidemiology should be persuaded to be isolated at home, and those with symptoms should be diagnosed and treated promptly. Encourage hand hygiene and respiratory courtesy to escorts and visitors.

25.6.9 *Medical imaging department*

On receiving the examination notification of suspected cases, the triage staff of imaging departments should inform technicians promptly. Technicians should wear level II protective equipment and lay disposable medical bedsheets to completely cover the inspection table. Patients shall be escorted to special rooms by designated staff for examination and assisted to remove the radiation protection equipment after the examination, and finally escorted back. It should be checked during the procedure whether patients are wearing standard surgical masks. After adopting level II protection, workers should disinfect the surfaces and air in inspection rooms.

25.6.10 *Central sterile supply department (CSSD)*

For disinfection of COVID-19 related reusable medical devices, the devices should be pre-treated on-site: Remove the heavy contaminants with flowing water first, then immerse with disinfectant-containing enzyme solution according to instructions; or soak in disinfectant containing 1000 mg/L of active chlorine for more than 30 minutes. For devices in contact with the patients' blood or body fluids, the active chlorine (bromine) concentration should be increased to 10000 mg/L. Then rinse the disinfectant with running water and wipe dry. Place them in special closed containers marked "Novel Coronavirus", to be collected by CSSD.

25.6.11 *Sampling, transferring and laboratory testing of clinical specimens*

Perform level II protection when collecting blood samples, and perform level III protection when collecting upper and lower respiratory samples. Put the collected samples into a disposable transparent sealed specimen bag (with biosafety mark), and deliver to the transfer person after no leakage is confirmed. The transfer personnel should wear surgical gown, disposable medical cap, medical surgical mask, and latex gloves. Wipe and sterilize the outer surface of the specimen bag with 75% ethanol, then put the bag into another new disposable transparent sealed specimen bag, and finally into the special specimen sealed transfer box labeled as "Novel Coronavirus"; Sterilize the surface of the transfer box with 75% ethanol. Keep the specimen upright during transportation and avoid jolts.

Laboratory workers should take level III protection, and wear disposable medical caps, medical protective masks, protective gown coveralls, goggles or protective face shields, first layer latex gloves, leak-proof wear-resistant boot covers, and second-layer latex gloves. Open the sealed specimen bag of the specimen in the biological safety cabinet; perform centrifuging in the fume cupboard, and the specimen is taken out after the centrifuge stops for 10 minutes. Any experiment that may generate aerosols should be performed in a biological safety cabinet. Handle medical waste and clean and disinfect the laboratory environment and the surface of objects according to regulations.

25.6.12 *Management of medical waste*

Dispose of infectious and pathological medical waste in double-layer medical waste packaging bags, and put injurious medical waste in sharps boxes. Medical waste should be packaged in accordance with "Provisions on the Standards and Warning Marks of Special Packages and Containers of Medical Wastes" and sealed effectively. Add a pressure-resistant hard carton to the outermost layer of the package and seal; it is absolutely forbidden to open it after sealing. A red "biohazard" sign should be printed on the surface of the carton, and the specific dimensions and specifications of the carton are not greater than 400mm × 300mm × 360mm. A yellow medical waste packaging bag should be placed outside the carton and temporarily placed at the place where the waste is generated. Appointed personnel should be responsible for the handover, and they should notify the solid recycling center to come for recycling, fill out the transfer order separately, and establish a ledger. Clean the ground surface of the temporary storage site and disinfect it with a disinfectant containing 1000 mg/L of active chlorine.

25.6.13 *Management of medical sewage*

The sewage generated during the epidemic should be controlled according to the sewage standards of infectious diseases medical institutions, and sterilization and disinfection should be strengthened to ensure that various indicators such as effluent fecal coliforms meet the requirements of "Discharge standard of water pollutants for medical organizations". Strengthen the control and management of wastewater and sludge discharge in sewage treatment stations to prevent the transfer of pathogens in different media. Sewage treatment projects located indoors must be provided with forced ventilation; equip staff with emergency supplies such as work clothes, gloves, and goggles; strengthen the monitoring and evaluation of the water quality of treatment facility discharge outlets and unit sewage outfalls. For departments with sewage treatment facilities, strengthen process control and operation management to ensure compliance with discharge standards; for departments without sewage treatment facilities, refer to the "Technical guidelines for hospital sewage treatment" and "Technical specifications for hospital sewage treatment" to construct temporary sewage treatment tanks (boxes) according to local conditions. Disinfect the sewage with liquid chlorine, chlorine dioxide, sodium chlorate, bleaching powder or bleaching essence, ozone, etc. Hospital sludge should comply with hazardous waste disposal requirements and be handled centrally by units with hazardous waste disposal qualifications.

25.6.14 *Postmortem disinfection*

The trained staff shall adopt level III protection, wearing work clothes, disposable medical caps, powered air-purifying respirators, medical protective gown coveralls, latex gloves, long-sleeved thick rubber gloves, and shoe covers. Use a disinfectant containing 3000–5000 mg/L of active chlorine or 0.5% peroxyacetic acid cotton balls or gauze to fill the patient's open channels or wounds, such as mouth, nose, ears, anus, and tracheotomy. Wrap the body using a double-layer sheet wetted with a disinfectant solution containing active chlorine (bromine) 3000 mg/L or 0.5% peroxyacetic acid solution, and seal the body in an impermeable double-layer body bag. If relatives agree to cremate the body, contact the funeral home to pick up the body as soon as possible, and indicate in the handover form of the body that the sanitary and anti-epidemic treatment has been carried out and the body needs to be cremated immediately. If relatives refuse to show up or refuse to transfer the body, medical institutions and funeral home shall try to persuade the relatives. If persuasion is ineffective, the medical institution should sign the body transfer form and then hand over the body to a funeral home for cremation directly.

Chapter 26
Biosafety Guidance for Pathogenic Biology Laboratories

Based on current knowledge of the biological, epidemiological, and clinical features of SARS-CoV-2, National Health Commission (NHC) of China issued *Laboratory Testing Guidelines for COVID-19 (4ᵗʰ edition)* that clarifies SARS-CoV-2 is temporarily classified as a category-B pathogenic microorganism based on its hazard level. Specifically speaking, there are different levels of safety precautions for different experiment operations. Before conducting experiments on live virus, laboratories need the approval of NHC to be eligible.

26.1 Viral Culture

Experiments involving virus isolation, culture, titration and neutralization, live virus and its protein purification, virus freeze-drying, and live virus recombination, are required to be conducted in biological safety level-3 (BSL-3) lab cabinets. Experiments involving nucleic acid extraction of viral culture and addition of splitting agents or inactivating agents should also be carried out in BSL-3 labs with protective conditions. Operations after the addition of splitting agents or inactivating agents can follow the instructions of safety protection level in Part III.

26.2 Experimental Operations on Animal Infection

Experiments on animal infection of live virus, sampling of infected animals, disposal and tests of infected samples, special examination of infected animals, and disposal of infected animal wastes are supposed to be conducted in biosafety cabinets of BSL-3 labs.

26.3 Experimental Operations on Uncultured Infectious Materials

If experiments are conducted on uncultured infectious materials including viral antigen detection tests, serological tests, nucleic acid extraction, biochemical analysis, and clinical samples before reliable inactivation, operations should be conducted in BSL-2 labs with self-protection measures of BSL-3 labs adopted.

26.4 Experimental Operations of Inactivating Agents

Experiments including viral antigen detection tests, serological tests, nucleic acid extraction, and biochemical analysis before the reliable inactivation of infectious microorganisms or live virus, should be conducted in BSL-2 labs. Experiments like molecular cloning that do not involve pathogenic viruses can be carried out in BSL-1 labs.

References

1. Chen W, Wang Q, Li YQ, *et al.* An overview of containment strategy in early stage of COVID-19 in China. *Chin Prevent Med.* 2020;54(3):239–244.
2. Ministry of Health of People's Republic of China. Guidelines on the Protection of Medical Staff in SARS Treatment (trial). *Chin J Nursing.* 2003;(07):4.
3. National Health Commission of the People's Republic of China. Notice of General Office of NHC on the Issuance of *Guidelines on the Use of Common Medical Protective Equipment in Prevention and Control of*

COVID-19 (trial). (2020-01-26) [2020-02-22]. http://www.nhc.gov. cn/yzygj/s7659/202001/e71c5de925a64eafbe1ce790debab5c6. shtml.

4. National Health Commission of the People's Republic of China. Notice of General Office of NHC on the Issuance of *Technical Guidelines on Prevention and Control of Novel Coronavirus Infection in Medical Institutions (1ˢᵗ ed).* (2020-01-22) [2020-02-22]. http://www.nhc.gov. cn/zhengce/zhengceku/2020-01/23/content_5471857.htm.

5. Shanghai Municipal Center for Disease Control and Prevention. Notice on the Issuance of *Requirement on the Use of Central Air-conditioning Ventilation System for the Prevention and Control of COVID-19 in Shanghai.* (2020-02-04) [2020-02-22]. http://wsjkw.sh.gov.ch/jbfk2 /20200218/1fc550dfd349487b92494fd79c434f07.html.

6. Shanghai Infection Control and Prevention Center. Notice on the Issuance of *Guidelines on Nosocomial Infection Control in Shanghai during COVID-19 Outbreak* (1ˢᵗ ed). (2020-02-19) [2020-02-22]. http:// www.sicpc.org/nd.jsp?id=189#_np=2_305.

7. Ministry of Ecology and Environment of the People's Republic of China. Notice on *Regulations of Medical Sewage and Urban Sewage Management During the COVID-19 Outbreak* (2020-02-01) [2020-02-02]. http://www.mee.gov.cn/zhengce/zhengceku/2020-02/02/ content_5472997.html.

8. Ministry of Ecology and Environment of the People's Republic of China. Notice of the Issuance of *Management and Technical Guidelines on Medical Wastes Disposal Solutions for Emergency Response During the Outbreak of COVID-19(trial).* (2020-01-28) [2020-02-22]. http: // www/gov.cn/xinwen/2020-01/29/content_5472997.html.

9. Epidemiology Group of COVID-19 Emergency Response Mechanism of Chinese Center for Disease Control and Prevention. Epidemiological feature analysis of COVID-19 [J]. *Chin J Epidemiol.* 2020;41(2):145–151.

10. Ministry of Health of the People's Republic of China. Technical Specifications on Hospital Isolation. *Chin J Nosocomiol.* 2009;19(13):1612–1616.

11. Expert Panel for COVID-19 Control and Prevention of Chinese Preventive Medicine Association. Latest knowledge of epidemiological features of COVID-19. *Chin J Epidemiol.* 2020;41(2):139–144.

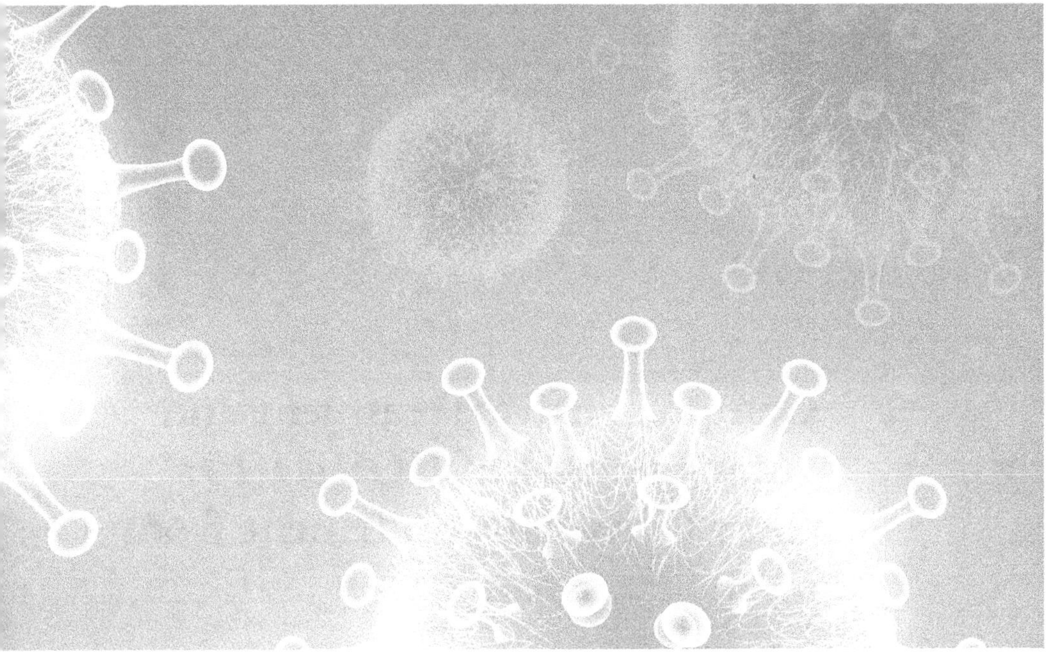

Appendix

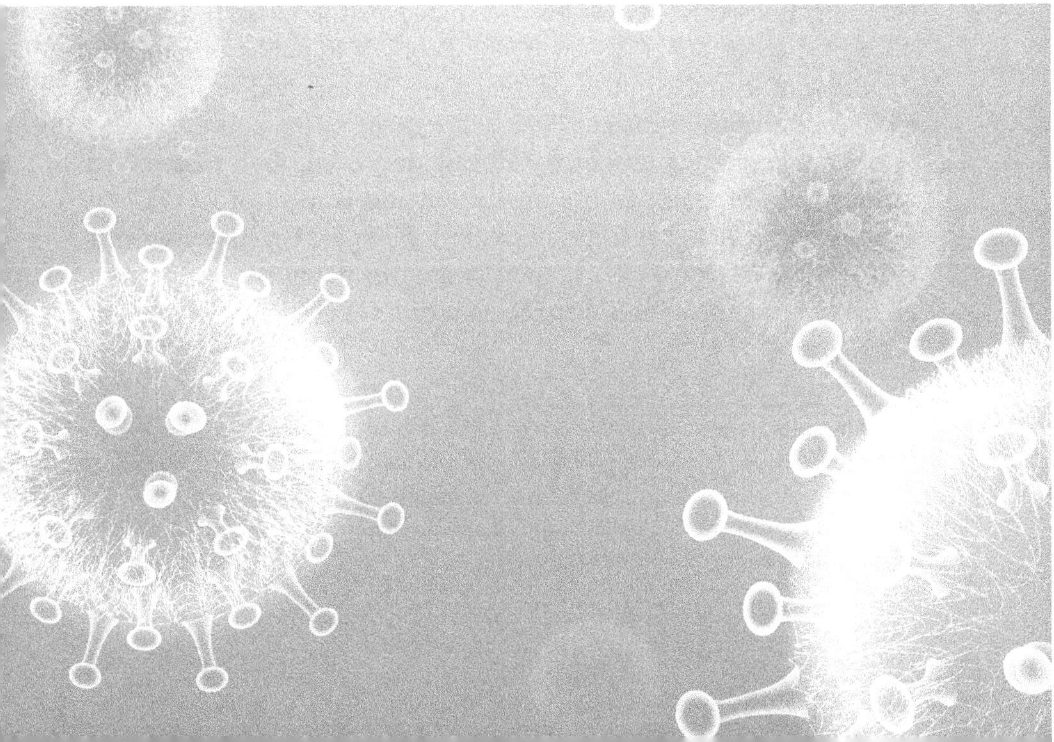

Comprehensive Treatment and Management of COVID-19: Expert Consensus Statement from Shanghai

Shanghai Clinical Treatment Expert Group for Coronavirus Disease 2019

Coronavirus disease 2019 (COVID-19) was first reported in Wuhan, Hubei province on December 31, 2019.[1,2] COVID-19, as a respiratory infectious disease, has been included in the Class B infectious diseases stipulated in the Law of the People's Republic of China on the Prevention and Control of Infectious Diseases and managed as a Class A infectious disease.

As the understanding of the disease deepened, the experience of various parts of China in the prevention and control of COVID-19 accumulated. Shanghai Clinical Treatment Expert Group for coronavirus disease 2019 issued an expert consensus statement on the comprehensive treatment and management of COVID-19.

Corresponding authors:
Wenhong Zhang, Department of Infectious Diseases, Huashan Hospital Affiliated to Fudan University, China. Email: zhangwenhong@fudan.edu.cn;
Hongzhou Lu, Shanghai Public Health Clinical Center, Fudan University, Shanghai, China. Email: luhongzhou@fudan.edu.cn

This consensus statement followed the China Novel Coronavirus Pneumonia Diagnosis and Treatment Guideline and further detailed parts of it,[3] incorporating domestic and foreign experience. Based on the continuous optimization and refinement of the treatment protocol, the aims of the consensus statement included improving clinical prognosis, reducing the patient's mortality rate, preventing the progression of the disease, and lowering the proportion of patients with severe illness.

Through early detection and quarantine of patients, comprehensive testing by the Center for Disease Control and Prevention, and active screening of close contacts, Shanghai managed to cut off the transmission chain and control the spread of the epidemic at its early stage. For mild patients, the focus of the consensus is mainly on the early detection, close monitoring, and timely intervention to prevent the patient from progressing to severe cases. For severe patients, the key during treatment lies in the adequate and prompt respiratory support, and close surveillance and refined treatment of the patient's multiple organ functions. As of March 21, 2029, 339 local cases were detected and there has been no new local cases for 19 consecutive days. Only four cases were reported dead so far and no medical staff infection was observed. We write this consensus in the hope that by sharing the experience of Shanghai clinical treatment expert group, we could enable more clinical physicians to comprehend the diseases and provide help to those in need.

1. Etiology and Epidemiological Characteristics

2019 novel coronavirus (2019-nCoV) is a new coronavirus belonging to the genus *Betacoronavirus*. On February 11, 2020, the International Committee on Taxonomy of Viruses (ICTV) named the virus severe acute respiratory syndrome coronavirus 2 (SARS-CoV-2).[4] Patients with COVID-19 and asymptomatic infection can transmit 2019-nCoV. Respiratory droplet transmission is the main route of transmission and it can also be transmitted through contact. There is the risk of aerosol transmission in confined enclosed spaces. 2019-nCoV can be detected in COVID-19 patients' stool, urine, and blood; some patients can still test positive for fecal pathogenic nucleic acid after the pathogenic nucleic acid test of respiratory specimens is negative. The population is generally susceptible. Children and infants can also develop the disease, but their condition is relatively mild.

2. Clinical Characteristics and Diagnostics

2.1 *Clinical characteristics*

The incubation period is 1–14 days, mostly 3–7 days, with an average of 6.4 days. Fever, fatigue, and dry cough are the main manifestations. It may be accompanied by runny nose, sore throat, chest tightness, vomiting and diarrhea. Some patients have mild symptoms, while a few have no symptoms or pneumonia.

The elderly and those suffering from diabetes, hypertension, coronary atherosclerotic heart disease, extreme obesity and other basic diseases are prone to develop severe conditions after infection. Some patients developed dyspnea one week after the onset of the disease, and the severe cases could progress to acute respiratory distress syndrome (ARDS) and multiple organ function damage. The interval of progression to severe course was around 8.5 days. It should be noted that some severe or critical patients only suffered low to moderate fever, or even normal temperature. The prognosis of most patients is good, and the death cases are mostly seen in the elderly and those with chronic underlying diseases.

Early CT examination of the lung usually showed multiple small patches or ground glass opacities especially in the outside area, with grid-like thickening in the inner veins. After a few days, the lesions increased and expanded to bilateral extensive, multiple ground glass shadows or infiltrating lesions, some of which could develop into consolidation. Broncho inflation sign was usually seen and pleural effusion was rare. A few patients progressed rapidly, and the imaging changes peaked on the 7–10th day. Typical "white lung" manifestations are rare. After entering the recovery period, the lesions were reduced and narrowed, and exudative lesions were absorbed. Fibrous cord shadow appeared and some of them could be completely absorbed.

In the early stage of the disease, leukocytes in peripheral blood was normal or decreased, and the number of lymphocytes was decreased. Liver function abnormality could appear in some patients, with increased level of lactic dehydrogenase (LDH), myozyme, myoglobin, and troponin. C-reactive protein (CRP) and erythrocyte sedimentation rate (ESR) increased in most patients while the procalcitonin was normal. Elevated level of D-dimer appeared in some severe cases, with changes of other coagulation indexes and increased lactate. Peripheral blood lymphocytes and CD4+ T lymphocytes decreased progressively. Electrolyte disorder, acid-base imbalance and metabolic alkalosis were common. The level of inflammatory cytokines (such as IL-6, IL-8, etc.) can be increased in the stage of disease progression.[5]

2.2 *Diagnostic criteria*

(1) *Suspect cases*

The suspect cases should be diagnosed through assessing both the epidemiological histories and clinical manifestations. Patients who satisfy any one of the epidemiological exposure histories as well as any two of the clinical manifestations can be diagnosed as suspect cases.

(i) Epidemiological history: Travel or residence in Wuhan and its surrounding areas or other communities with cases reported within 14 days before the patient's symptom onset; a contact history with patients (positive results of nucleic acid test of SARS-CoV-2) within 14 days before the patient's symptom onset; a contact history with patients with fever or respiratory symptoms from Wuhan and its surrounding areas, or the communities with cases reported within 14 days before the patient's symptom onset; and clustering of cases.

(ii) Clinical manifestations: Fever and/or respiratory symptoms; radiological features of pneumonia described above; normal or decreased total white blood cell count, and a decreased lymphocyte count in the early stage of the disease.

(2) *Confirmed cases*

The suspected cases with one of the following etiological evidence can be diagnosed as confirmed cases.

(i) A positive result of nucleic acid test of SARS-CoV-2 by real-time fluorescence RT-PCR; (ii) the virus gene sequence is highly homologous to the known SARS-CoV-2; (iii) positive nucleic acid test of SARS-CoV-2 in sputum and in lower respiratory tract secretion of patients with tracheal intubation.

2.3 *Differential diagnosis*

COVID-19 should be distinguished from viral pneumonia caused by other known viruses, including influenza virus, parainfluenza virus, adenovirus, respiratory syncytial virus, rhinovirus, human metapneumovirus, severe acute respiratory syndrome (SARS) coronavirus, etc. It should also be distinguished from pneumonia caused by *Mycoplasma pneumoniae*, *Chlamydia pneumonia* and other bacteria. In addition, differentiation from non-infectious diseases such as vasculitis, dermatomyositis, and organizing pneumonia should also be performed.[6,7]

2.4 *Clinical classifications*

(1) *Mild cases*

The clinical symptoms are mild and no pneumonia manifestation can be found in imaging.

(2) *Ordinary cases*

Patients have symptoms like fever and respiratory tract symptoms, and pneumonia manifestation can be seen in imaging.

Attentions should be paid to the early signs of deterioration for ordinary cases. Based on current clinical studies, the elderly (>65 years) with underlying diseases, CD4+ T lymphocyte count <250/μL, significantly increased blood IL-6 levels, significant radiological progress

>50% within 2 to 3 days, lactic dehydrogenase (LDH) >2 times the upper limit of normal value, blood lactic acid ≥3 mmol/L, metabolic alkalosis, etc. are all early warning indicators of severe disease.

(3) *Severe cases*

Meet any of the following: (i) respiratory distress, RR≥30 breaths/min; (ii) oxygen saturation is less than 93% at rest state; (iii) arterial partial pressure of oxygen (PaO_2)/ fraction of inspired oxygen (FiO_2) ≤300 mmHg (1 mmHg = 0.133 kPa). For high altitude areas (above 1000 meter), PaO_2/FiO_2 values should be adjusted based on equation of PaO_2/FiO×[Atmospheric Pressure (mmHg)/760].

Patients with radiological progress >50% within 24–48 hours should be treated as severe cases.

(4) *Critical cases*

Meet any of the following: (i) respiratory failure occurs and mechanical ventilation is required; (ii) shock occurs; and (iii) complicated with other organ failure that requires monitoring and treatment in ICU.

2.5 *Clinical evaluation*

The patient's symptoms, signs, fluid volume, gastrointestinal function and mental state should be closely monitored every day. All patients should be dynamically monitored for terminal blood oxygen saturation. For severe and critical cases, timely blood gas analysis should be performed according to the changes of the patient's condition; blood routine, electrolytes, CRP, procalcitonin, LDH, blood coagulation function indicators, blood lactic acid, etc. should be tested at least once every 2 days; liver function, kidney function, ESR, IL-6, IL-8, and lymphocyte subsets, should be tested at least once every 3 days; and pulmonary radiological examination usually should be evaluated every 2 days. For patients with ARDS, routine ultrasound examination of the heart and lungs at the bedside is recommended to observe extravascular lung water and cardiac parameters. For monitoring of extracorporeal membrane oxygenation (ECMO) patients, refer to the implementation section of ECMO.

3. Treatment

3.1 *Antiviral treatment*

Hydroxychloroquine sulfate or chloroquine phosphate can be tried as oral administration, as well the nebulization and inhalation of interferon. It is not recommended to use three or more antivirals at the same time. As soon as the viral nucleic acid is not detected, the antiviral treatment should be stopped. The efficacy of all antiviral drugs remains to be evaluated in further clinical studies.

The plasma from convalescent patients can be tried on severe and critical cases with positive viral nucleic acid results. The detailed operation and management of adverse reactions should be carried out according to the "Clinical Treatment Program for Recovery of New Coronary Pneumonia Patients in Recovery Period (Trial Version)".[8] It is more effective to be infused within 14 days upon disease onset. If the viral nucleic acid is continuously detected at the later stage of the disease, the plasma treatment of convalescent patients can also be tried.

3.2 *Treatment of mild and ordinary patients*

It is necessary to strengthen supportive treatment to ensure sufficient calorie intake; pay attention to the balance of water and electrolytes, maintain the stability of the internal environment, and closely monitor the vital signs and oxygen saturation of patients. Effective oxygen therapy should be given in time. In principle, antibiotics and glucocorticoids are not used routinely. It is necessary to closely observe the changes of the patient's condition. If there is significant development with a risk of becoming serious, it is recommended that comprehensive measures be taken to prevent the disease from progressing to severe, and low-dose short-term corticosteroids can be used cautiously as appropriate (for the specific plan, see section on the application of glucocorticoids). Heparin anticoagulation and high-dose vitamin C therapy are recommended.[9,10] Low molecular weight heparin (LMWH) lasted for 1 to 2 doses per day until the level of D-dimer returned to normal. Once the fibrinogen degradation product (FDP) ≥10 µg/mL and/or D-dimer ≥5 µg/mL, unfractionated heparin was used for anticoagulation. High dose of vitamin C was given by intravenous drip of 100 mg/kg/day for ordinary patients, and the duration of use was aimed at a significant improvement in oxygenation index. If there is a progression of pulmonary lesions, it is recommended to use high-dose broad-spectrum protease inhibitor ulinastatin until the lung imaging examination is improved. In the event of a "cytokine storm", intermittent short-term veno-venous hemofiltration (ISVVH) is recommended.[11]

3.3 *Treatment of organ function support for severe and critical patients*

(1) *Protection and maintenance of circulatory function*

Implement the early active principle of controlled rehydration. It is recommended to evaluate the effective volume and initiate fluid therapy as soon as possible after admission. Severe patients can choose intravenous or fluid resuscitation via colon according to the conditions. Lactic acid Ringer's solution is the first choice for replenishing liquids. With regard to vasoactive drugs, norepinephrine combined with dopamine is recommended to maintain vascular tension and increase cardiac output. For patients with shock, norepinephrine is the first choice. It is recommended that low-dose vasoactive drugs should be used at the same time as fluid resuscitation to maintain circulatory stability and avoid excessive fluid infusion. It is recommended that drugs are used to protect the heart; and sedatives harmful to the heart are avoided as far as possible in severe and critical patients. For patients with sinus bradycardia, isoproterenol can be used. It is suggested that for patients with sinus rhythm, heart rate <50 beats/min, and hemodynamic instability, low dose of isoproterenol or dopamine should be used to maintain the heart rate at about 80 beats/min.

(2) *Reduce pulmonary interstitial inflammation*

Severe pulmonary interstitial lesions caused by COVID-19 can lead to deterioration of lung function, so a large dose of broad-spectrum protease inhibitor ulinastatin is recommended.

(3) *Protection of renal function*

Appropriate anticoagulant therapy and appropriate fluid therapy are recommended as soon as possible. See the section on the prevention and treatment of "cytokine storm", and the section on the protection and maintenance of circulatory function.

(4) *Protection of intestinal function*

Prebiotics can be used to improve the intestinal microecology of patients. Use raw rhubarb (15 20g plus 150 ml boiled water) or Dachengqi decoction orally, or enema every day for 5–7 days.

(5) *Nutritional support*

Enteral nutrition is the first choice, by nasal feeding or jejunal approach. The nutritional preparation of whole protein is the first choice, with 25–35kcal/kg (1 kcal = 4.184 kJ) of energy per day.

(6) *Prevention and treatment of "cytokine storm"*

High-dose intravenous vitamin C (HIVC) and unfractionated heparin for anticoagulation are recommended. High doses of vitamin C were injected intravenously with 100–200 mg/kg/d. The goal of continuous use is to significantly improve the oxygenation index. High-dose broad-spectrum protease inhibitor ulinastatin is recommended to be given at 1.6 million units per 8 hours, which can be reduced to 1 million units per day when oxygenation index > 300 mmHg under mechanical ventilation. Anticoagulation therapy can be used to protect endothelial cells and reduce the release of cytokines. When FDP is more than 10 µg/mL and/or D dimer is more than 5 µg/mL, unfractionated heparin (3–15 IU/kg per hour) is given intravenously. The coagulation function and platelets must be reexamined 4 hours after the onset of heparin and the appropriate dose is obtained by using titration method for the reduction of FDP and D-dimer. ISVVH for 6–10 hours per day is not used until the cytokine storm is ameliorated.

(7) *Sedation muscle relaxation and artificial hibernation therapy*

Patients who are mechanically ventilated or receive ECMO should be sedated on the basis of analgesia. For patients with serious man–machine resistance in the establishment of artificial airway, short-term use of low-dose muscle relaxants is recommended. It is suggested that severe patients with oxygenation index <200 mmHg should use hibernation therapy. Artificial hibernation therapy can reduce metabolism and oxygen consumption, dilate pulmonary vessels and significantly improve oxygenation. Continuous intravenous injection is recommended, and patients' blood pressure should be closely monitored. Use opioids and dexmedetomidine with caution. It can lead to abdominal distension due to the increased level of IL-6 in critical patients, so opioids should be avoided to prevent aggravation of abdominal distension. As COVID-19 can also inhibit the function of sinoatrial node and sinus bradycardia, sedatives that can inhibit the heart should be used with caution. To prevent the occurrence and aggravation of pulmonary infection, prolonged excessive sedation is avoided, and muscle relaxants should be withdrawn as soon as possible. It is recommended to closely monitor the depth of sedation.

(8) *Oxygen therapy and respiratory support*

(i) Nasal cannula or mask oxygen inhalation: SaO_2 ≤93% while breathing air or SaO_2 <90% after activities, or 200 mmHg <PaO_2/FiO_2 < 300 mmHg, with or without respiratory distress, continuous oxygen therapy is recommended.

(ii) High-flow nasal cannula (HFNC) oxygen therapy: If respiratory distress symptom is not improved or getting worse, or PaO_2/FiO_2

is between 150 and 200 mmHg after nasal cannula or mask oxygen inhalation 1–2 hours, high flow nasal cannula should be considered.

(iii) Noninvasive positive pressure ventilation (NPPV): Failure to respond to high-flow nasal cannula oxygen, or 150 mmHg < PaO_2/FiO_2 < 200 mmHg after HFNC 1–2 hours may require consideration for NPPV.

(iv) Invasive mechanical ventilation: If respiratory distress symptom is not improved or getting worse or PaO_2/FiO_2 <150 mmHg after HFNC or NPPV 1–2 hours, invasive mechanical ventilation should be considered. Mechanical ventilation using lower tidal volumes plus positive end-expiratory pressure (4–8 ml/kg predicted body weight) is a preferred protective ventilatory strategy.

(9) *Extracorporeal membrane oxygenation (ECMO) support for COVID-19 patients with refractory hypoxia despite lung protective ventilation*

<u>Indications and Intervention Timing</u>
Following the standardized treatment process of ARDS with lung protective ventilation, optimizing PPEP, combined with neuromuscular blocking agents, recruitment maneuvers, and prone positioning, the patients still presented with (i) PaO_2/FiO_2 <100 mmHg and/or (ii) arterial pH <7.25 with $PaCO_2$ ≥60 mmHg for 6 hours, ECMO support will be indicated. In case of any of the following, salvage ECMO shall be established immediately: (i) PaO_2/FiO_2 <50 mmHg for >1 hour; (ii) PaO_2/FiO_2<80 mmHg for > 2 hours; or (iii) uncompensated respiratory acidosis pH <7.2 for > 1 hour.

<u>ECMO mode and vascular access</u>
V-V mode is preferred even with hypoxic hemodynamic disturbance. Percutaneous V-V access by femoral and jugular veins with two cannulas has more advantages as it offers fast setup and reliability in a stressful environment. Considering that the increase of intraperitoneal pressure in patients with COVID-19 may interfere with ECMO

blood flow, the tip of the drainage (femoral) cannula can be placed into the right atrium for 1 cm despite more recirculation.

<u>ECMO management special for COVID-19</u>
Keep hemoglobin >11 g/dl and $DO_2/VO_2 > 3$ is recommended to allow some reserve as the target of oxygenation. Ultra-lung-protective ventilation is preferred during ECMO. Avoid the temptation to turn up the ventilator settings or FiO_2 above rest settings during V-V support. It is necessary to control excessive spontaneous respiration to avoid aggravating lung injury so be very careful in evaluating whether patients can tolerate Awake ECMO. Anticoagulation management should be strengthened to deal with the common hypercoagulation risk.

<u>ECMO weaning and trail-off</u>
When ECC support is less than 30% of total, native lung function may be adequate to allow coming off ECLS, and a trail-off is indicated by clamping sweep gas of ECMO on vent rest settings PSV or spontaneous breathing at 50% FiO_2 if meet all of the following conditions for 24–48 hours: (i) hemodynamics are stable; (ii) lung radiograph along with EIT and ultrasound examination improvement; (iii) P/F >150mmHg, PCO_2 ≤50mmHg and RR ≤20; (iv) temperature <38°C; (v) Murray Score 2–3; and (vi) Hct >35%.

3.4 *Treatment of organ function support for severe and critical patients*

(1) *Corticosteroids*

Use corticosteroids with caution. Corticosteroids can be administered to patients with significant radiological procession or signs/symptoms of severe cases (i.e., SaO_2 ≤93% at rest state without oxygen inhalation, respiratory distress with RR≥30 breaths/min, or oxygenation index≤00 mmHg). Corticosteroids are indicated for patients with acceleration of disease progression and patients at risk of intubation. Corticosteroids should be withdrawn promptly in patients with intubation or ECMO when blood oxygen concentration is effectively maintained. For non-severe patients, the recommended dose of methylprednisolone is 20–40 mg/d, while 40–80 mg/d for severe cases. The duration of corticosteroid treatment is recommended to be 3–6 days. The specific corticosteroid protocol can be adjusted according to body weight and condition of the patient.

(2) *Immunomodulatory medicine*

Subcutaneous injection of thymosin 2–3 times a week has some effects on improving patients' immune function, preventing the disease from deterioration, and shortening the viral clearance. Due to the lack of specific antibodies, high-dose intravenous immunoglobulin therapy is currently not recommended. However, for some patients with low levels of lymphocytes and at risk of co-infection with other viruses, human immunoglobulin can be administered intravenously at 10 g/d for 3–5 days.

(3) *Precise diagnosis and treatment for bacterial and fungal co-infection*

Perform clinical microbiological monitoring of all severe and critical cases. Sputum and urine should be collected daily for culture, and timely blood cultures are suggested for patients with a high temperature. All suspected sepsis patients with indwelling catheters should be examined simultaneously with peripheral venous blood culture and catheter blood culture. Also, all suspected sepsis patients may consider collecting peripheral blood for molecular diagnostic examination of etiology, including molecular diagnostic tests based on PCR and next-generation sequencing.

Elevated levels of procalcitonin are suggestive for the diagnosis of sepsis/septic shock. CRP is increased in patients with COVID-19 when the disease is aggravated, while its specificity is not enough for diagnosing sepsis caused by bacterial and fungal infections.

Critical patients with opened airway who received invasive airway management are prone to have bacterial and fungal infections in the later stages of disease. If sepsis occurs, empirical antimicrobial treatment should be given as soon as possible. For patients with septic shock, a combination of empirical antibiotics covering the most common Enterobacteriaceae, Staphylococcus and Enterococcal infections simultaneously should be used prior to etiological examinations. The beta-lactamase inhibitor complex may be chosen for patients with hospital-acquired infections. If the treatment response is poor or the patient has severe septic shock, carbapenems can be used instead.

If patients are considered to have Enterococcus and Staphylococcal infections, glycopeptide antibiotics (vancomycin) can be used to undertake empirical treatment. For bloodstream infection and pulmonary infection, Daptomycin and Linezolid can be taken into consideration respectively. For catheter-related infections in critical patients, the empirical treatment for these cases should cover methicillin-resistant Staphylococcus. Glycopeptide antibiotics (vancomycin) can be selected for empirical treatment. Candida infection is common in criticalpatients and should be empirically covered in treatment when necessary. Echinocandin anti-fungal drugs can be useful as well. With the extended length of hospitalization of critical patients, drug-resistant infections have gradually increased. At this time, the use of anti-bacterial drugs must be adjusted according to drug sensitivity tests.

(4) *Prevention and control of nosocomial infection*

According to "The Basic System For Prevention and Control of Infection in Medical Institutions (Trial Version)" issued by the National Health Commission in 2019, evidence-based infection prevention and control intervention strategies were actively implemented to effectively prevent ventilator-related pneumonia, intravascular catheter-related bloodstream infection, catheter-related urinary tract infection, carbapenem-resistant gram-negative bacilli, and other multi-drug-resistant bacteria or fungi infection. Head of bed, oral care with chlorhexidine every 2–6 hours and continuous suction of secretion above the air bag were performed to prevent ventilator-related pneumonia. Catheter-related bloodstream infection was prevented with chlorhexidine skin disinfection, with chlorhexidine-containing film and alcohol cotton tablet for catheter interface disinfection in severe cases.

Measures against multidrug-resistant bacteria in severe patients included special personnel care, chlorhexidine skin disinfection, CRE active screening, one-time isolation gowns, strict disinfection of the environment, and disinfection of the specialized equipment.

"Guidelines on Prevention and Control of Novel Coronavirus in Medical Institutions (First Edition)", "Guidelines on the Use of Common Medical Protective Equipment in the Prevention and Control of Novel Coronavirus Pneumonia (Trial Version)", and "Guidelines for the Medical Personal Protection Techniques during Novel Coronavirus Infection (Trial Version)" issued by the National Health Commission were strictly followed in the process of strengthening management. First, qualified and standardized process design were needed, including doctor–patient access, medical personnel access, etc. Second, appropriate personal protective equipment should be used: medical personnel who contact suspected or diagnosed patients should wear medical protective masks, isolation gowns, goggles or visors, double-layer gloves, double-layer shoe covers, etc.; comprehensive masks or positive pressure breathing masks are recommended when aerosol can easily spread across short distance. Finally, the implementation of various disinfection and isolation measures should be strictly carried out, including the use of negative pressure ward as far as possible, the use of hydrogen peroxide to disinfect the environment at least once every 4 hours and to wipe the surface of objects, and the use of hydrogen peroxide to disinfect the environment at the end. Through various prevention and control measures, the risk of nosocomial infection can be minimized and novel coronavirus nosocomial infection in medical personnel can be eliminated.

(5) *Management of children with COVID-19*

All pediatric suspect cases are required to be isolated at the hospital until they are ruled out as having SARS-CoV-2 infection based on the negative results of nucleic acid testing for SARS-CoV-2 on two respiratory samples collected at least 24 hours apart. Clinical assessment of the severity of the disease is necessary before an appropriate treatment regimen can be decided. Non-severe COVID-19 is usually self-limited and symptomatic treatment is recommended. In the meantime, close observation is extremely important for children who have either non-severe symptomatic or asymptomatic infection as the disease can worsen within 5–8 days after onset, based on the clinical findings of COVID-19 in adults. For severe and critical COVID-19 pediatric patients, timely supportive care and monitoring is the mainstay of the treatment regimen and pediatricians may refer to the adult protocol. Empirical antibiotic initiation is not routinely recommended for treatment of SARS-CoV-2-associated pneumonia without evidence of super bacterial infection. Given that no evidence has shown current available antiviral agents to be effective for COVID-19 and that their potential adverse effects are a concern in children, antiviral agents should not be routinely recommended for the treatment of COVID-19 at this stage, although antiviral agents including lopinavir, arbidol, ribavirin, and α-interferon inhalation have been tried as part of the treatment of COVID-19 in adults. So far, the effect of these antivirals on COVID-19 is not clear and they are still under clinical evaluation. For the treatment of severe COVID-19, ribavirin could be considered because it is often used in pediatric patients in China and severe adverse events have rarely been reported. The use of Chinese traditional medicine depends on the child's compliance with taking medicine, although national treatment protocol recommends the combined use of Western and Chinese traditional medicines. In addition, influenza virus screening is necessary to rule out possible co-infection and to avoid unnecessary empirical overuse of oseltamivir.

All close contacts should be strictly quarantined and closely monitored for symptoms for 14 days after last contact with the infected person, and COVID-19 should be evaluated once symptoms develop. Based on clinical observations, the nucleic acids of SARS-CoV-2 in nasopharyngeal/throat swabs are undetectable within 6–25 days after illness onset. Of particular attention, the nucleic acids of SARS-CoV-2 are frequently detected in stool samples from pediatric patients with mild COVID-19, and the virus shedding phase in feces could last for at least 2 weeks and even exceed 1 month. Thus, standard hand hygiene should be strictly implemented during close contact with an infected child at the convalescent stage.

3.5 *Integration of traditional Chinese and Western medicine treatment*

Additional traditional Chinese medicine improves the treatment effect for COVID-19 patients. The specific schemes should be according to the diseases condition, local climate characteristics, and different patients' physical conditions.

3.6 *Discharge standards*

Patients meeting all the following standards can be discharged: (i) normal body temperature for more than 3 days; (ii) significantly recovered respiratory symptoms; (iii) pulmonary radiological examination shows obvious absorption and recovery of acute exudative lesion; (iv) negative results of nucleic acid tests of SARS-CoV-2 for two consecutive times (sampling interval at least 1 day apart); (v) negative results of nucleic acid tests of SARS-CoV-2 in stool sample after viral clearance in respiratory samples; and (vi) total course of disease is over 2 weeks.

3.7 *Health management of discharged patients*

(1) For discharged patients, close follow-up is still required. Follow-up is recommended from 2–4 weeks after discharge to the designated follow-up clinic.

(2) When a patient is discharged from the hospital, his/her place of residence and address in the city should be specified.

(3) Patients should rest at home for 2 weeks after discharge from the hospital, avoid activities in public places, and must wear masks when going out.

(4) Follow-up should be conducted by local medical institution assigned by the district health committee according to the patient's address (including a room in hotel). Professionals will visit the patient's residence for follow-up of body temperature and health status twice a day for 2 weeks, and give relevant education.

(5) If fever and/or respiratory symptoms recur, the corresponding medical institution shall report to the District Health Committee and the District Centers for Disease Control and Prevention in time, and assist in sending them to the designated medical institutions in the area for treatment.

(6) After receiving the report, the District Health Committee and the District Centers for Disease Control and Prevention should report to the higher-level division in a timely manner.

References

1. Health commission of Wuhan city. Reports on the current situation of unknown origin pneumonia in Wuhan city. (2020-12-31) [2020-02-25]. http://wjw.wuhan.gov.cn/front/web/showDetail/2019123108989.

2. World Health Organization. Naming the coronavirus disease (COVID-2019) and the virus that causes it. [2020-02-25]. https://www.who.int/emergencies/diseases/novel-coronavirus-2019/technical-guidance/naming-the-coronavirus-disease-(covid-2019)-and-the-virus-that-causes-it.

3. National Health Commission of the People's Republic of China. The diagnosis and treatment of COVID-19 (6th edition). (2020-02-18) [2020-02-25]. http://www.nhc.gov.cn/yzygj/s7653p/202002/8334a8326dd94d329df351d7da8aefc2/files/b218cfeb1bc54639af227f922bf6b817.pdf.

4. Gorbalenya AE, Baker SC, Baric RS, *et al.* Severe acute respiratory syndrome-related coronavirus: the species and its viruses — a statement of the Coronavirus Study Group. *BioRxiv.* 2020 (2020-02-11) [2020-02-25]. https://www.biorxiv.org/content/10.1101/2020.02.07.937862v1.

5. Lu HZ, Ai JW, Shen YZ, *et al.* A descriptive study of the impact of diseases control and prevention on the epidemics dynamics and clinical features of SARS-CoV-2 outbreak in Shanghai, lessons learned for metropolis epidemics prevention. *medRxiv.* 2020 (2020-02-23) [2020-02-25]. https://www.medrxiv.org/content/10.1101/2020.02.19.20025031v1.

6. Ai JW, Zhang Y, Zhang HC, *et al.* Era of molecular diagnosis for pathogen identification of unexplained pneumonia, lessons to be learned. *Emerg Microbes Infect.* 2020; In press.

7. Ai JW, Zhang HC, Xu T, *et al.* Optimizing diagnostic strategy for novel coronavirus pneumonia, a multi-center study in Eastern China. *medRxiv.*

2020 (2020-02-17) [2020-02-25]. https://www.medrxiv.org/content/ 10.1101/2020.02.13.20022673v1.

8. Wang D, Hu B, Hu C, *et al.* Clinical characteristics of 138 hospitalized patients with 2019 novel coronavirus-infected pneumonia in Wuhan, China. *JAMA.* February 07, 2020. https://jamanetwork.com/journals/ jama/fullarticle/2761044.

9. Chen Y, Ma L, Song X, *et al.* Beneficial effects of fluid resuscitation via the rectum on hemodynamic disorders and multiple organ injuries in an experimental severe acute pancreatitis model. *Pancreatol.* 2015;15(6):626–634. DOI: 10.1016/j.pan.2015.09.001.

10. Ma L, Chen Y, Song X, *et al.* Vitamin C attenuates hemorrhagic hypotension induced epithelial-dendritic cell transformation in rat intestines by maintaining GSK-3β activity and E-cadherin expression. *Shock.* 2016;45(1):55–64. DOI: 10.1097/SHK.0000000000000486.

11. Li L, Tang YQ, Mao EQ, *et al.* Mechanism of hemofiltration in treatment of severe acute pancreatitis. *World Chin J Digestol.* 2004;12(12):2822– 2825. DOI: 10.3969/j.issn.1009-3079.2004.12.012.

12. Shang L, Zhao J, Hu Y, *et al.* On the use of corticosteroids for 2019-nCoV pneumonia. *Lancet.* (2020-02-11) [2020-02-25]. DOI:10.1016/ S0140-6736(20)30361-5.

13. National Health Commission of the People's Republic of China. Basic system of infection prevention and control in medical institutions (Trial Version). (2019-05-18) [2020-02-25]. http://www.nhc.gov.cn/yzygj/ s7659/201905/d831719a5ebf450f991ce47baf944829.shtml.

14. National Health Commission of the People's Republic of China. Technical guidelines for the prevention and control of novel coronavirus infections in medical institutions (1st ed). (2020-01-22) [2020-02-25]. http://www.nhc.gov.cn/yzygj/s7659/202001/b91fdab7c304431 eb082d67847d27e14.shtml.

15. National Health Commission of the People's Republic of China. Guidelines on the use scope of common medical protective equipment in the prevention and control of novel coronavirus pneumonia (Trial Version). (2020-01-26) [2020-02-25]. http://www.nhc.gov.cn/yzygj/ s7659/202001/e71c5de925a64eafbe1ce790debab5c6.shtml.

16. National Health Commission of the People's Republic of China. Technical Guidelines for the Protection of Medical Staff during the COVID-19 epidemics (Trial Version). (2020-02-21) [2020-02-25]. http://www. henanyz.com/uploadAttach/20200224/20200224095242_338.pdf.

Translators' Afterword

The year 2020 will be imprinted on the memories of many of us owing to the coronavirus outbreak. For most of the people in China during the early stage of the epidemic, it felt like someone pressed the "pause" button on their regular lives.

Since the SARS epidemic, renowned experts in public health, epidemiology, and infectious diseases worldwide have continually warned about the dangers of the next emerging respiratory disease capable of causing a pandemic. On January 18, 2020, a couple of days before China officially announced sustained interpersonal transmissive capability of the novel coronavirus, Professor Zhang Wenhong was giving a speech in Beijing on influenza, advising the public to prepare for the next influenza outbreak. "Life has never been naturally quiet and peaceful, but there has always been someone safeguarding you," said Prof. Zhang during the speech. Later that day, he returned to Shanghai and immediately started to lead the fight against COVID-19 at his affiliated hospital — Huashan Hospital.

The experts, like Prof. Zhang, are fighting at two fronts simultaneously: one front involves directly facing the invisible enemy, SARS-CoV-2, and the other is confronting the spread of misinformation and disinformation about COVID-19. The WHO describes the second front as fighting of the "infodemic." Prof. Zhang's methods of disseminating information through humor — although always maintaining sincerity — during speeches and interviews about the epidemic, led to his rapid popularity in China as one of the prominent figures communicating the science to the public. The information he promotes is practical, to-the-point, and expressed with clarity while maintaining a disposition of professionalism.

As a clinical expert, Prof. Zhang led the team at Huashan Hospital in composing this book: *COVID-19 — From Basics to Clinical Practice*. It was published by Fudan University Press in April and rapidly became one of the most authoritative and influential medical works on the studies of COVID-19 in response to the epidemic. At the time of the publication, the situation of China's epidemic control was turning into a positive trend, while the outbreaks continued to spread in other countries. The outbreaks even showed growing trends of further deterioration in countries like Italy, Spain, the United Kingdom, France, Germany, the US, Iran, Japan, and South Korea. With a heart of humanistic love, Prof. Zhang gifted the copyright of the book and authorized Fudan University Press for further licensing of the overseas copyrights for free. He hoped to share China's experience gained during the fight against COVID-19 to the international society through publications of the translations of this book and to promote global solidarity in the battle against the pandemic.

Being given the generous gift by Prof. Zhang while facing the pandemic, Fudan University Press felt the urgent need to summon translator talents for rapid translations of the book into multiple languages at the earliest possible time. The Department of Copyright of the Press was facing a daunting test to accomplish this task. On the afternoon of March 27, 2020, Mr. Zhang Yongbin, the Deputy Chief Editor responsible for copyright licensing, called for a meeting with the persons in charge of the Medical Branch, the Department of Copyright, and the Department of Publicity to discuss on the matter. It was decided on the meeting to issue a recruitment order globally to attract volunteers with translation skills in various languages. The order was officially released through the WeChat social media account of the Press and quickly attracted widespread attention in the society. The news was reported by more than 100 significant media, including Xinhua News Agency, People's Daily, Guangming Daily, and China Daily, with over 66 million reads on the Internet. As of March 31,

2020, only four days after the news release, the Press received 606 application emails with trial translations from applicants worldwide. Among the trial translations, there were 209 in English, 37 in Spanish, 30 in French, as well as the ones in Italian, German, Persian, Russian, Portuguese, Japanese, Korean, and Romanian.

Since the numbers of translation talents and trial translations were the most abundant for English, the Press initiated the translation work for this language first. On the afternoon of April 2, 2020, the Department of Copyright of the Press invited senior English editors Lin Xianghua and Cao Zhenfen to review the trial translations in their spare time during the Qingming Festival holiday. They performed anonymous reviews on the 209 trial translations and selected 28 for further evaluations. On the afternoon of April 7, 2020, the Press handed over the 28 trial translations to the Huashan Hospital team led by Professor Zhang Wenhong for final reviews. Eventually, the team chose 13 translators with a professional background in biology, medicine, or English linguistics. The Press organized for a collaborative translation work dividing the 26 chapters of the book into two chapters for each translator. The English translation team was officially assembled through the creation of the WeChat group on April 9, 2020.

The 13 members of the translation team are Wang Xun, Cheng Xiaoheng, Qin Zhizhen, Yuan Rongjie, Cheng Siyuan, Ding Ruoyu, Li Haiqi, Luo Chuqiao, Nie Yao, Xin Chao, Xue Bing, Yang Xuejiao, and Zhang Yi.

In addition to the 13 translators, the WeChat group also included the First Deputy Chief Editor, Dr. Wang Xinyu, and the Editorial Secretary, Dr. Liu Qihui, from the author team of the original book; the Editor from World Scientific Publishing, Xiao Ling; the Deputy Chief Editor, Zhang Yongbin, the Deputy Director of the Medical Branch, Wei Lan, the Project Director of the Department of Copyright, Dai Wenqin, and the Copyright Editor, Wang Hui, from Fudan University Press. During the translation work, the translators consulted the authors of the original book, the Chinese editors, the English editors, and the copyright editors for questions and got answers promptly. The close interactions and communications guaranteed the high efficiency of the translation process.

After the completion of the translation drafts by the translators, to ensure the quality of the translation, the Press divided the translation team into three groups for cross-proofreading by the group leaders. Cheng Xiaoheng, the leader of group one, was responsible for chapters 1 to 9; Qin Zhizhen, the leader of group two, was responsible for chapters 10 to 17; and Yuan Rongjie, the leader of group three, was responsible for chapters 18 to 26.

When the revisions by the group leaders were concluded, Wang Xun subsequently performed overall proofreading of the whole book. Eventually, four managing editors from the Huashan Hospital team, Wang Xinyu, Jin Jialin, Chen Jiazhen, and Xu Bin, performed the last reviews and finalized the manuscript.

We summarized the entire translation process here in detail to record such a brand-new attempt during a particular time.

The translation work of this book was completed smoothly, on schedule, and with high quality. It was achieved with a meticulous organization by the Press, selfless efforts from the 13 translators around the clock, the final review by the team led by Professor Zhang Wenhong, as well as the dedication of countless colleagues and friends. Due to space limitations, we are unable to list all the names one by one. We would like to express our high respect and sincere gratitude to everyone from all walks of life who cared, supported, and participated in this translation work.

Due to the time limitations and various linguistic levels of the translation team, mistakes and errors are inevitable. We welcome all corrections and suggestions from the readers for improvements in the translation for future editions.

The pandemic of COVID-19 poses a daunting challenge to every country on the planet. We hope to achieve the vision for global solidarity in the battle against COVID-19 through the rapid sharing of information and experience on the disease.

Finally, as written in some of the chapters in the book, we hope for early accomplishments in developing drugs, therapies, and vaccines against SARS-CoV-2. We believe that after this costly lesson, people around the globe will have a more profound understanding that we all belong to a community with a shared future.

A brighter tomorrow and a prosperous future await a more united humanity.

Fudan University Press,
together with the translation team
May 5, 2020